Tension

CRITICAL GLOBAL HEALTH: *Evidence, Efficacy, Ethnography*
A series edited by Vincanne Adams and João Biehl

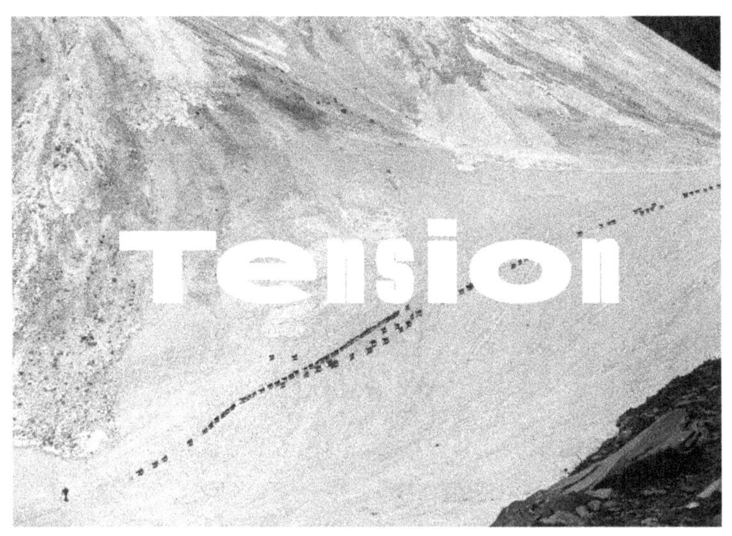

Mental Distress and Embodied Inequality in the Western Himalayas

NIKITA KAUR SIMPSON

Duke University Press *Durham and London* 2026

Project Editor: Liz Smith
Cover designed by Matthew Tauch
Typeset in Garamond Premier Pro by Westchester Publishing Services

Library of Congress Cataloging-in-Publication Data
Names: Simpson, Nikita Kaur, [date] author
Title: Tension : mental distress and embodied inequality in the Western Himalayas / Nikita Kaur Simpson.
Other titles: Critical global health
Description: Durham : Duke University Press, 2026. | Series: Critical global health: evidence, efficacy, ethnography | Includes bibliographical references and index.
Identifiers: LCCN 2025033422 (print)
LCCN 2025033423 (ebook)
ISBN 9781478033295 (paperback)
ISBN 9781478029830 (hardcover)
ISBN 9781478062042 (ebook)
Subjects: LCSH: Gaddis (Indic people)—Social life and customs | Gaddis (Indic people)—Mental health | Social change—India—Himachal Pradesh | Social change—Health aspects—India—Himachal Pradesh | Economic development—Social aspects—India—Himachal Pradesh | Economic development—Health aspects—India—Himachal Pradesh
Classification: LCC DS432.G275 S484 2026 (print) | LCC DS432.G275 (ebook) | DDC 306.0954—dc23/eng/20251117
LC record available at https://lccn.loc.gov/2025033422
LC ebook record available at https://lccn.loc.gov/2025033423

Frontispiece: A flock coming down from Sach Pass. Spring migration from the Chamba side of the Dhaula Dhar to Chandrabhaga Valley. Photograph by Christina Noble, 1979.

Cover art: Soujanyaa Boruah, *CloudsRollingUp*. Courtesy of the artist.

For Avtar and Pritpal, who brought me here,
And Shyam and Soujanyaa, who found me.

Hathe goai hinde hadna aaye

You try to whistle back that which you
let slip from your hand.

—GADDI PROVERB

Contents

Author's Note

Throughout this book, most place-names have been changed, with the exception of cities such as Dharamsala and districts such as Kangra and Chamba. All names are pseudonyms, and many accounts have had defining characteristics altered or excised to protect the anonymity of those with whom I spoke. Field notes and accounts have also been anonymized and sometimes cut into multiple accounts.

Fieldwork for this book was conducted in Gaddi dialect, Hindi, and English. I have refrained from using any conventional style for the transliteration of phrases or words. I have used identifiable English-language spellings for words from Hindi and Gaddi that appear frequently, as well as for individuals, places, names, deities, and institutions.

Even when speaking Gaddi or Hindi, my interlocutors consistently used the English word *tension* when speaking of their distress. I italicize this term and also the term *BP* throughout to remind the reader that I'm using these words with their local meanings, not their standard English meanings.

The stories within may be distressing for some readers. They include accounts of death, sexual abuse, rape, violence, and severe mental illness. Readers who may be triggered by these accounts are encouraged to exercise care.

This book includes accounts of some individuals who are now deceased, and permission has been sought from their relatives to tell their stories, where appropriate. All photographs taken by the author were taken with the permission of those who feature within them.

Preface: A Mother's Body

The first time my mother collapsed, we were on a summer holiday. I remember her dark skin quivering before her legs buckled. Her blood pressure had skyrocketed so high, my father said, that she could have had a stroke. On that summer's day, we were crammed into a room that overlooked an Italian lake, an operatic backdrop to the scene. It happened while she was fighting with her sister, and the wind was so strong that it almost drowned out their voices. It took her five long minutes to come around. My aunt stroked her hair.

I have always thought of my mother's body as consubstantial with my own. I have never known how to articulate our mutuality, an unknowing that propels me. Her skin is my skin; together we are exposed to the world. Through her touch, she absorbs her children's worries. Our excesses are held in her fascia and joints, causing them to become stiff. As her body has fallen apart, I have always felt that it was because of me, because of us.

She lost her first tooth after she breastfed me. Leached of calcium, the hard enamel crumbled like cheese. She lost three more, one with each child. She mostly laughs about the holes now, but sometimes I catch her grimacing as she tongues the gummy flesh in the back of her mouth.

My mother is a pediatric geneticist. She diagnoses tiny babies born with abnormalities, infants who begin seizing as they enter the world. She works with parents who have had one, two, three children with the same catastrophic illnesses. What is the loss of a few teeth in comparison? she always says. But these babies take a bit of her too. She goes to the funerals of all of those who don't survive.

Her bones followed her teeth, becoming brittle and fragile. She first felt the pain when she, my brother, and I were visiting my aunt in London. I must have been eleven, and my brother nine. While my aunt was at work, my mother took us to Hyde Park to go horse riding. It was May, and the park was dense with life, but the air was chilly and entered my mother's bones. It never left.

My mother was diagnosed with rheumatoid arthritis, or a general atopic autoimmune connective tissue disorder. But a lot of her pains aren't captured by this label. Especially the parts related to care.

It got worse around the time that my grandparents were in a car accident. I was in my first year of university, fifteen thousand kilometers away. They were picking my brother up from school, and my grandfather pushed the accelerator instead of the brake. My grandmother broke eleven ribs, and her lung collapsed. My mother slept with her in the hospital until she could come home, then watched every day as she blew into a little machine that made a ball float. It was meant to show that her lungs were strengthening, but I always felt like it was my mother's strength that held the ball in the air.

My mother's body is a weathervane. She can divine a great storm coming from subtle changes in moisture and heat in the atmosphere. Somehow, her body is more porous, more permeable than others—maybe from all those years of care. Things were bad one summer, as La Niña washed over Australia's east coast, bringing the wettest summer on record. When I woke up in London, I could sense her level of pain by reading the weather forecast in Sydney.

When the pain gets too much, she asks my sister to sit on her legs. The compression, she says, gives her some relief. Hot masala tea also helps, and fizzy water. I had these ready for her when she came to visit me when I was doing my fieldwork, high up in the foothills of the Indian Himalayas. She thought she was coming to look after me again, to give me a break from the stories I was hearing day after day about distress and illness. I thought that her pain had nothing to do with these stories of distress and illness. But, unlike the women in these stories, when my mother arrived, her body slowed, her joints released. She slept in, I made her tea, and she would sit in our kitchen as we sliced vegetables and made *dal*-rice. She rested, for a moment.

I BEGIN THIS BOOK with my mother's body because it is where I first encountered the slippery ways in which distress accumulates across generations and crosses from atmospheres and relations into joints, bones, and flesh. Through her endless acts of care and listening, of cleaning and feeding, she holds her parents, her sister, her children, and her patients. But this takes something from her. These acts are life-affirming, but they are also depleting. I saw the same dynamic in almost every woman, and many men, whom I encountered during my fieldwork in rural North India between 2017 and 2019 with people from the Gaddi community. Their bodies held vast networks of relationships and absorbed the distress of intimate others from past and present. But this act of holding relations left their bodies wrecked and their minds wracked. Until I arrived in the foothills of the Himalayas, I didn't think there was a word for this kind of relational distress. Until I encountered *tension*.

Introduction

WHAT IS *TENSION*?

Dev Bhumi

To get up into the mountains, we always took the road through the slate mines. This used to be a road that snaked from the village into the mines, out of which trucks brought trailers full of well-trimmed slates. The road was built with the financing of Mr. Robert Barkley Shaw, a British investor who commenced mining operations in 1867 through the establishment of the Kangra Valley Slate Company. For a time, Shaw's road made the surrounding Pahari villages rich; some say they were "the richest villages in all of South Asia." But now the road crumbles every monsoon season when the river rises and brings down debris from explosions upstream. The result is a wound in the ancient hills—kilometers of rugged slates, huge slabs, and tiny chips piled into human-made mountains that you must scramble up and down to get to the tree line. The slates crunch under your feet, and you slide and tumble down with them. The trick is to remain

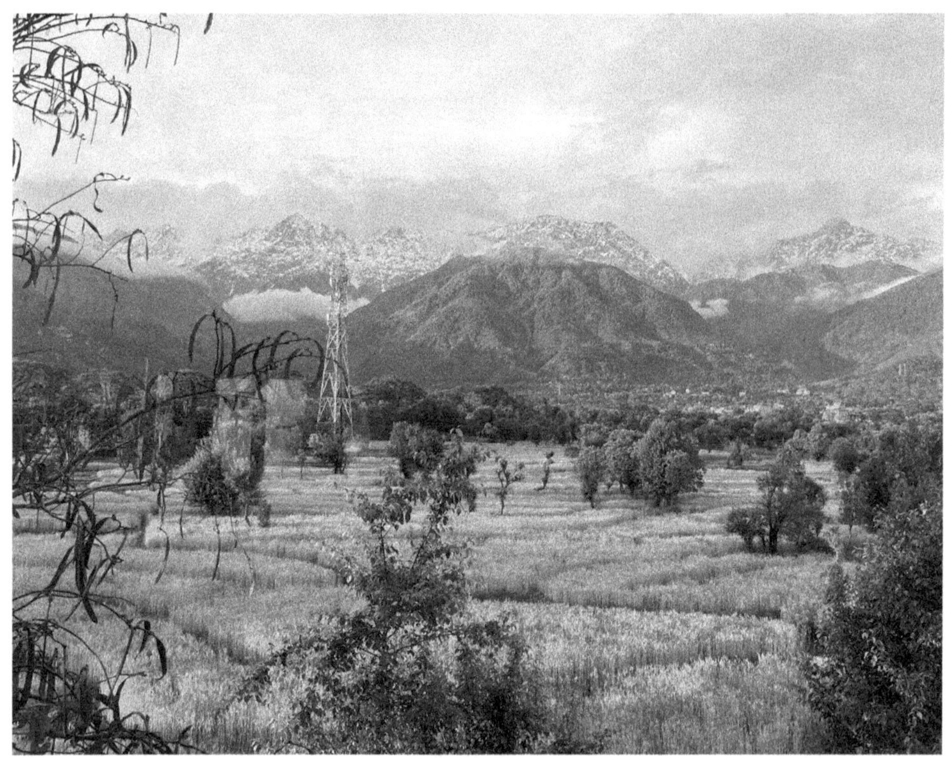

FIGURE I.1. The Dhaula Dhar mountains at dusk, taken from the plains below. Photograph by Nikita Kaur Simpson, 2024.

nimble, moving your weight from one foot to another so that the push of your foot is equivalent to the push back of the slates. It is different from the way you navigate hill walking.

Once when we were crossing from the road onto the slates, Shankar—my Gaddi research companion—caught my arm. He pointed across the ravine to a cavern that lay just under a cliff in the adjacent mountain. My eyes, weakened by years of close reading, couldn't follow his line of sight and kept circling the spot. But finally, I saw it—a dark streak of blood—brownish against the orange of the cut rock. Around the streak a number of tiny dark dots circled, vultures with wingspans longer than a human is tall. A horse had died—injured and then killed while carrying packs of slate on its back along the high mountain road from the mine to the yard in the nearby village where it is sold. Its death was so silent, up there high on the ridge, the birds' calls lost against the sound of the explosions that shake the valley.

The mining is illegal now, outlawed years ago in a Shimla court hundreds of miles away by civil servants who sought environmental protection. This ruling came after most of the Gaddi men had given up their herds, and the mines had ruined their pastures. Besides, there is still demand for slate from all the city dwellers who are building homes in the lower foothills, escaping the heat and smog of the plains. So the men keep returning, seeking a blessing from Saloti Mata, the goddess of slate, to protect them from government closure as well as the frequent landslides that can bury a man whole.

After you cross the slate mountains, the sun's glare disappears, and you enter a canopy of rhododendron trees, which, before the monsoon, paint the hill a deep cerise. Their flowers can be collected and ground with coriander and salt to make a delicious chutney, but if left to rot, they make the path slick with pink mucus that can prove as dangerous as the slates to the unseasoned traveler. Shankar was rhythmic as he climbed these hills—years of herding sheep and goats up and down the mountain were present in his gait. Now he must walk more slowly, shepherding only hikers and day-trippers. Walking beside him, I became aware of the pressure I put on my thighs to haul myself up the mountain, jolting and forcing my form. His thin frame was erect despite his heavy pack. Shankar wore Decathlon hiking boots like his clients, but most Gaddis climb the mountain in plastic shoes, loafers bought for a hundred rupees in the market. Shankar told me these were the most comfortable choice.

Whenever we walked these trails, up toward his family's shepherding hut, Shankar pointed out places where he had experienced uncanny encounters with ghosts, witches, and Nepali gangs searching for medicinal plants. The thick canopy was home to the Jungle Raja, an incubus who comes to women in their sleep, luring them into illicit sexual forays. It also provided cover for *churel*, the ghosts of infertile women or those who die in childbirth. They appear to exhausted shepherds or miners as beautiful maidens, tempting them, before revealing themselves as old hags with sagging breasts and pockmarked skin, sucking what is left of their victim's vitality. This forest is also the site of a great war in August each year, on one night during the monsoon rains. On this night all the witches in the area congregate and channel their black magic by lifting their dresses and taunting the gods. The Indra Nag, a manifestation of Lord Shiva, meets them in battle. If the witches win, there will be no rain, and famine and misfortune will plague the Gaddis for the following year. If the Indra Nag wins and the witches are defeated, rain will pelt down in the following days and for weeks to come, and a year of abundance and fortune will ensue.[1]

These dark forces are unknown to the foreigners who come seeking shelter in these hills. Instead, Kangra has been a site of conflict and relief for invading armies, weary pilgrims, and exiled governments for centuries. It has hosted Muslim, Sikh, Hindu, Christian, and Buddhist rulers, soldiers, monks, and courtesans over the past five hundred years. This history is rich, complex, and violent: The Islamic Mughal ruler Akbar captured the region in the 1566, before the Sikh king Jai Singh took it back and gave it to the Hindu Rajput king Sansar Chand in 1785. It was the site of conflict between the Gurkhas and Sikhs through the latter part of the eighteenth century, before being recaptured by Ranjit Singh in 1809. Singh granted the Rajput Katoch kings feudal lordship, and they built a thriving courtly culture that patronized artists and pastoralists alike until the First Anglo-Sikh War of 1846. Quelling a series of revolts, the East India Company annexed Punjab and brought Kangra under the rule of the British administration in Lahore.

The "wild and picturesque scenery" of the Dhaula Dhar—the Himalayan mountain range in which Dharamsala is nestled—formed a subsidiary military cantonment for British troops stationed at Kangra and was first occupied by a "Native regiment" that was being raised in the area. They established residences on a "plot of waste land, upon which stood an old Hindu resthouse or *dharamsala*, whence the name adopted for the new cantonment."[2] From the annexation of Punjab in 1849 until the catastrophic earthquake of 1905, European houses and officers' barracks were established along the steep paths of the hillside—first to house British and "Native" military families, the Sixty-Sixth Gurkha Light Infantry, and then an increasing population of civilians who were attracted to the "pine-clad mountain side," the "luxuriant Kangra valley . . . [a] picture of rural quiet," and the burgeoning trading post that supplied goods to the "European residents, officials and their servants."[3] The hill station became a ghost town following the earthquake that destroyed the majority of buildings in the upper cantonment. It left only the Anglican church—St. John in the Wilderness—which hosted a monument to James Bruce, Eighth Earl of Elgin and viceroy of India, who had died there in 1863.

After Indian independence in 1947, Kangra and Dharamsala remained part of the now-divided province of Punjab and hosted large national military cantonments on the lower Dhaula Dhar slopes. After the Fourteenth Dalai Lama fled Tibet in 1959, Prime Minister Jawaharlal Nehru offered the upper hill settlements of McLeod Ganj to the Dalai Lama's exiled government. This led to the resettlement of more than fifteen thousand Tibetan refugees and the construction of Tsuglagkhang—the Dalai Lama's main temple in McLeod Ganj—and a number of monasteries, Tibetan medical hospitals, libraries, and schools in the surrounding hills. The teachings of the Dalai Lama have attracted a flow of international visitors and devotees since the 1960s. Many of those who came some three or four decades ago—to learn yoga and meditation, *thangka* painting, and tai chi—have never left. Instead, they bought plots of cheap agricultural land on which they built vast homes, social development organizations, and therapeutic practices. Their houses have hosted salons for Indian and European intellectuals, folklorists, architects, philosophers, and writers.[4]

Today a new kind of digital nomad is drawn to the vistas, the Himalayan marijuana, and small bars along the trail. Some come for a visit, journaling and sipping tea in any one of the vegan cafés, before they move on to Rishikesh or Manali. Others stay longer—renting a room in one of the guesthouses. Many escapees became my companions along my journey—an octogenarian psychoanalyst practicing from a mud house in the village, a designer who was setting up a forest school, two software engineers who devoted themselves to building accessible technologies for the village children. I suppose I was one such person, though I came to follow distress rather than seek relief from it along the mountain trails.

FOR THE GADDI PEOPLE, the imagined potencies of cosmopolitan Dharamsala pale in comparison to the majestic deities that are said to have inhabited this place for much longer. As for many Himalayan residents from Uttarakhand to Arunachal Pradesh, many Gaddis do not think of the Dhaula Dhar as a series of peaks but rather as a divine plateau marked by a set of passes. They call it Dev Bhumi—the land of the gods, or literally "god earth," a place the divine inhabit in peace without the disturbance of humans.[5] It is there, on the snowcapped plateau, that Lord Shiva resides, grieving for his beloved consort Parvati. Shankar told me this great love story during one of our trips up to the shepherding hut. We sat around the hearth, picking at corncobs blackened on the coals. "Gorji," Shankar began, using Parvati's Gaddi name, "always worshipped Dhundu [Lord Shiva], even when he was a sadhu [ascetic]."

> She would go to his cave, clean it, and bring him fruit. But when she saw how dark [skinned] he was, she decided she didn't want to marry him. Dhundu came out of meditation and decided that he wanted to marry Gorji. He went to her [mother's brother] house (Himraj, the ruler of snow) and asked their family, "What gift do you want to marry me?" She said, "I don't want anything for my house, not utensils. I don't want sheep and goats for they will just be killed by leopards." He asked again. She told him that it was snow that she wanted, because a draft of snow would stop Dhundu from coming to take her back to his house and marrying

> her. When it was time for the *baraat* [marital procession], the whole sky was filled with stars. She woke in the night and saw the snow starting to fall. She was very happy.
>
> By the morning, everything was covered in snow. Shiva was on the other side of the mountain, waiting to go and pick up his bride. He was very worried. How would he go? He knew he had to unblock the road. He ordered elephants, then horses, to clear the route. But they could not pass. So he fashioned a Gaddi man and his herd from the snow. It was only this first Gaddi man who could clear the route. They were able to cross the passes. Gorji, back in her uncle's house, heard the instruments of the *baraat* playing. At last, Dhundu and his consort reached her house. Her friends called her, saying that her beloved Dhundu was in a bad way. She saw him, and still saw that he was ugly. She was very upset, but the marriage went ahead. As they began to walk around the fire, Dhundu transformed into his most beautiful form. But before the marriage ritual could end, Dhundu ran away. Gorji, now enchanted, followed him up Mount Kailash.
>
> Gorji couldn't find Dhundu. She was so hurt that she took her own life. When Dhundu saw her body, he was wracked by grief and anger. He began to dance with her body in his arms. The gravity of his dance caused the destruction of all that was. From under his feet, the Himalayas were born, and Gorji's body began to split into twelve parts. The pieces of her body fell across the land. Five of those parts fell in the Himalayan region, two in Kangra.

It is Dhundu's frantic dance, and the creative energy that emanated from Gorji's body, that is the animating principle of life and of time. Like Hindus across India, Gaddis also used Gorji's other name, Shakti, in this telling, and more generally to refer to an energizing principle without which there would be no motion.[6] According to elderly men and women, the Gaddis used to be the keepers of this place, the protectors of the mountains, of this life force, through their custodianship of the land. It was only a Gaddi who could clear the route for this mighty deity, who could facilitate this great and tempestuous love. It is through communion with land and with animals that they filled their own bodies with such vitality. But now only a few gnarled persons look back toward the passes. To others, being a custodian of Dev Bhumi means something very different. These others look the other way, toward the plains, toward a new threat that blocks this life force.

* * *

"*Tension* rolled in from the plains," Shankar's sister Anushka told me one day, as we sat overlooking the valley.

ONCE, FROM THAT VANTAGE point, you could expect to see right down to the military cantonment of Pathankot, some four hours' drive away. Now these clear days came only in a slice of October, when the September rains had washed away a year's worth of pollution, and before the Diwali firecrackers broke the sky. Of all districts in the Himachali hills, *tension* hit these villages on the Dhaula Dhar's southern foothills first, according to Anushka, for this was a fault line. Above these villages, the majesty of the mountains; below, the scourge of the plains. Indeed, many Gaddi people saw themselves as straddling this fault line. In their fields one could find both mango and fir trees. They enjoyed the rich meat of goats who fed on mountain herbs, and rice grown in the engorged paddies in the lowlands.

Living on this fault line is not new, for the Gaddi people had made their looping grazing route—from the high pastures of the Dhaula Dhar in their homeland of Chamba to the hot plains of Punjab—for centuries. However, in the past century they have experienced a rapid shift in livelihood, from agropastoralism to military or government service, or to waged work in the slate, tourism, hydropower, and construction sectors. The enclosure of land, increasing urbanization, and the creep of noxious lantana weeds into grazing pastures has made shepherding unfeasible. The sweaty hardship of a nomadic life is less appealing to young men, and no one wants to marry a shepherd.

This shift in livelihood has altered the intimate life of this community and their relations of care. The Gaddi house, formerly crafted from mud and dung, is now made of cold concrete. It is inhabited by a nuclear family and populated with new and modern appliances that elderly Gaddis don't know how to use. An educated bride is now desirable and is expected to channel her literacy into the future trajectories of her children, who are hopefully educated in the local private school and sent to Delhi or Chandigarh or Dubai after matriculation. Where grandmothers are one of thirteen children, mothers are one of four or five, and daughters want only one or two. A woman and her husband supposedly treat their son and their daughter equally, yet girl children are increasingly aborted, and young women are surveilled even more acutely than in the past as they step beyond the bounds of the house to attend school, college, or their job in a nongovernmental organization (NGO).

New forms of inequality in income, education, and status have deepened within and between Gaddi households. Where one brother is in the military, another runs a small corner shop. Where one neighbor sells his land to a hotelier, another remains a petty laborer on its construction site. These inequalities sometimes run along the existing social divides of caste but sometimes depart from them, allowing lower-caste Gaddis to aspire to higher-class status, and leaving higher-caste Gaddis struggling to maintain their prestige. The result is a fractured social hierarchy and a deeply unstable sense of tribal belonging.

Gaddiness itself has become, or perhaps always was, a fraught social identity—one that shifts in content and form depending on who is watching. The category of Gaddi came into being as a fixed and coherent identifier only through the classificatory gaze of anthropologist-administrators, like Cambridge anthropologist John Henry Hutton, in the 1931 census of India.[7] Without consistent criteria for the definition of a tribe (*jana*), tribalness came to be characterized by the practice of traditional religion or animism, and distinctively egalitarian ways of life that sat outside the hierarchical caste (*jati*) system.[8] In the gaze of the postcolonial state since 1947, this tribalness has taken on new meaning, signifying "backwardness" that warrants material uplift but retains social distinction. At the time, such Scheduled Tribe (ST) status was awarded only to Gaddis whose registered residence was over the other side of the Dhaula Dhar in Chamba. Kangra Gaddis resided in the state of Punjab, a place where it was thought that no backward people or tribes existed. From the formation of the state of Himachal Pradesh in 1966, upper-caste Gaddis have campaigned for ST status based on their landownership and kinship links to Gaddis in Chamba and their distinctive agropastoralist way of life—a status they were granted only in 2002. However, not all Gaddi-speaking people are recognized as ST—lower-caste Gaddis are recognized as Scheduled Caste (SC), and Gaddi-speaking Bhat Brahmins are classified as Other Backward Classes (OBC).[9] For ST Gaddis, such state recognition has come at the very moment when the distinctive Gaddi agropastoral way of life is less evident and when Gaddis of all castes are at pains to resignify their "backward" cultural practices against a newly muscular Hindu nation.[10] Shifts in economic prosperity mean that the door has swung open for Gaddi-speaking people whose families have never practiced shepherding to make claims to Gaddi respectability through the adoption of aesthetic practices—ways of dressing, dancing, worshipping, eating, drinking, and being intimate.[11]

It is in view of this wider aesthetic politics of respectability that people speak of the present as better than the past. The Gaddi people are no longer stigmatized as primitive or savage by neighboring communities or the state; they are wealthier, life is easier, and people are educated. "Life is better today," most Gaddi people told me. There is much less hard work to do, people are no longer poor (*garib*). "Women are "coming up," and "maximum" (most) people don't believe in caste anymore."[12] As Pinky Hota observes of tribal people across India, such material uplift is entwined with religious pedagogy in the present nationalist atmosphere.[13] Tribal people in the colonial state figured as exoticized, primitive Others. Postindependence affirmative action policies positioned them as backward subjects of development and as animists with a psychological disposition that involved "unalloyed satisfaction in the pleasures of the senses."[14] In both cases, tribes, as Virginius Xaxa writes, were racially and thus biopsychologically distinct—defined precisely by the fact that they were not "contaminated by Hindu civilization" and were said to "belong to either Negroid, Australoid, or Mongoloid stock, with nomadic habits and a love of dance and music."[15] In the present, the Gaddis, like other ST groups, seek a way out of the double bind that is posed by tribal recognition—that one could be recognized as tribal only if one admitted one's racial difference, one's savagery or backwardness. They seek a way of being distinctive and authentic, without being locked into a savage slot, excluded from either modernity or futurity. They are at pains to present themselves as respectable, autochthonous Hindus—distinct from both their proximate Tibetan, Gurkha, and even Central Indian migrant neighbors and the chimeric Muslim Other.[16]

In this time of progress, or perhaps issuing from it, a darker force had also raised its head. "People are following dark things these days" was a refrain I heard frequently. "People these days are terrified; there is more fear now than there has ever been." It is precisely in this moment of perceived prosperity that the forces of witchcraft, black magic, illness, and *tension* have risen. Indeed, modern time itself seemed to be signaled in the eyes of Gaddi people by the advent of *tension*. The condition evokes the loss of tradition, the depletion of the land, the loss of connection to animals, the breakdown of social relations. To some extent, this fraught present is attributed to the epoch of *kali yug*—the fourth and final stage of an endlessly repeated cycle of epochs, characterized by intensifying moral decay.[17] But deeper investigation revealed more proximate causes—in ruptured relationships, intergenerational conflict, economic insecurity, and ecological destruction. The rise of *tension* might be seen as the intimate experience, or perhaps the embodied cost, of this broader project of progress and respectability as it reworks the relations of the self to the other in domestic and neighborly worlds, as well as at broader national scales.

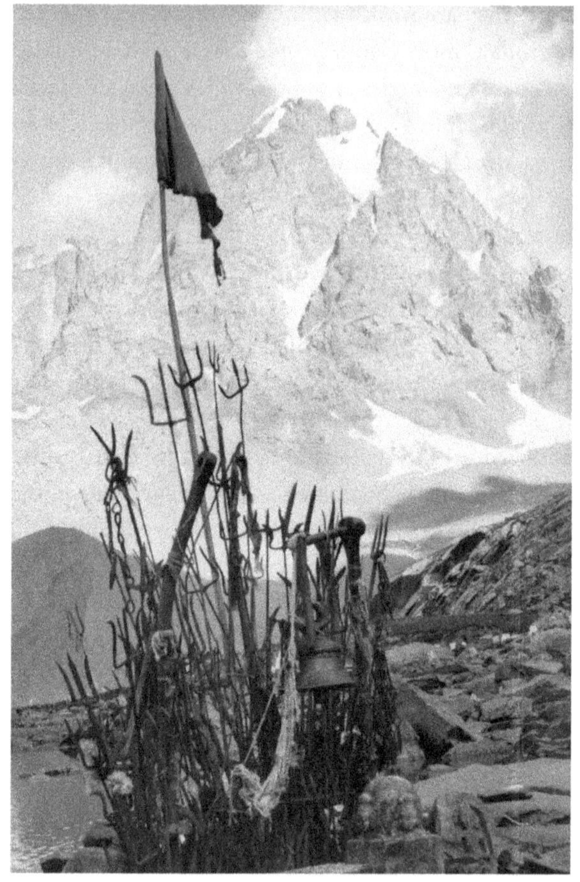

FIGURE I.2. Mount Kailash, Shiva's seat, and shrine to him at Manimahesh Lake, 13,000 feet. Photograph by Christina Noble, 1983, part of the collection held by Noble and the British Museum.

Following *Tension*

In Hindi, Punjabi, Urdu, and even Turkic languages, *tension* is a polysemic term, wielded in different ways to describe the strains and scrapes of life. In the Gaddi community, *tension* is used by people without noticing, an ordinary expression that one heard so often that it lost any particular poignancy. "No *tension*, madam," a taxi driver would reassure me after a near miss on the road. "She gives me so much *tension*," a mother would laugh, of a daughter who spilled the tea she was meant to place before a guest. Yet, as I came to be enfolded into the stresses of life during my fieldwork in the Dhaula Dhar foothills, a more visceral form of *tension* began to emerge.

Gaddi people used *tension* to speak to inherently ambiguous, capricious experiences of disorientation—as Sianne Ngai suggests, "what we might think of as a state of feeling vaguely 'unsettled' or 'confused.'"[18] *Tension* opened a window into the giddy moments when people aren't sure what to feel about the times they are in, or aren't sure what to feel with respect to intimate others, especially those of different generations. These feelings are different, as Danilyn Rutherford points out, from the prescribed sentiments that issue from social roles. Instead, they inhabit a gap between the social role and the fraught and awkward experience of social life.[19] There are other words in Gaddi dialect for sentiments that have stronger social scripts. The term *bhiog*, for instance, is used to express grief, particularly for a lover or partner; *berry*, to express the anger directed at a lover. *Rog* is used to express physical illness, like the Hindi term *bimar*, and *guttan* to express a feeling of suffocation, similar to that which is symptomatic of panic or anxiety. *Ghum*, borrowed from Urdu, is similar to the Hindi term *dukh*, used to express sorrow or sadness. However, none of these terms captures the same kind of distress or bodily symptoms held in the notion of *tension*, with its precise link to present conditions of uncertainty and aspiration. "There is no word for *tension* in Gaddi," I was told. I encountered *tension* in a whisper through gritted teeth while sitting side by side on a public bus, in an outburst in the privacy of an empty kitchen, or muffled by tears during a domestic altercation. During these encounters the sufferer would raise their head, uttering a familiar refrain, *Mujhe bahut tension hai* (I have so much *tension*). The space became laden with this *tension*. At its nadir, it was a slowly churning melancholy, but as they spoke of their sufferings, it whipped up into a buzzing anxiety. Through these encounters I came to realize that expressions of *tension* were not only speech acts with communicative functions. Instead, articulations of *tension* were fissures in the psychic fabric of the everyday—moments wherein their tellers sought new forms of voice.

Veena Das, in *Life and Words*, draws on the work of Stanley Cavell to distinguish between speech and voice. Reflecting on her own encounters with survivors of the India-Pakistan Partition living in Delhi, Das was struck by the ways in which experiencing violence renders subjects "voiceless—not in the sense that one does not have words—but that these words become frozen, numb, without life."[20] Such voicelessness is a state where one's access to context is lost, meaning that the everyday is rippling with a skepticism that manifests in affects of fear and anticipation. In the Gaddi case, there is no critical traumatic event that infuses the collective experience of the everyday. However, spending time among the Gaddi community, one is struck by the deeply fraught nature of the present—a skepticism that ripples below the surface of the everyday, generating affects of envy, fear, and distress. This comes from a different kind of loss of context, one that issues not from spectacular violence but from a fraying of the social fabrics—relations of caste, class, and tribal belonging—that shape this community and from an unraveling of the expectations of kinship, conjugality, and gender that undergird them. This is not to say that this context ever existed in any timeless or holistic form but, instead, that fractured relations of care across this community generate painful experiences of distress. Acts of telling *tension* work both to register these fractured care relations in the mind and body and to push back against the structural changes—to livelihood, land, nation, and religion—that drove them. Acts of telling *tension* were scalar moments where people spoke, through their bodies, to the embodied cost of social change.

For Das's sufferers in post-Partition Delhi, finding voice occurred "both within and outside the genres that become available in the descent into the everyday."[21] For the Gaddis, the genres through which these acts of telling occurred were quotidian and multiple. They included ambivalent somatic complaints of aches and pains, humoral imbalances—overheating and cooling, wind and dryness. They also included clipped, grieving, or angry expressions of strain in intimate—conjugal or affinal, neighborly or intergenerational—relations within and around the home. These acts of telling *tension* were charged not only through the language used to make them but also by the shared affects that met in bodies and places in states of atmospheric intensity. *Tension* was not experienced or expressed as an individual pathology.

Importantly, my interlocutors stressed that *tension* did not exist only in their bounded interior worlds, but neither did it exist only exterior to their bodies.[22] Instead, it seemed to emanate from the body; it mingled with the smoke from the fire, making my throat catch and my eyes water. *Tension* was an atmosphere that, as Michael Schnegg puts it, is both an objective ontological entity and an intersubjective experience. Atmospheres originate outside of the box of the psyche, or in between bodies. They are room-filling—soliciting everyone who enters, independent of how they relate to the situation when they enter.[23] To understand *tension*, it was essential to both register this objective entity and become part of it—to pick up on the "fleeting, subtle, and hardly discernible aspects of [people]'s lives," as Tine Gammeltoft writes, that are latent, diffuse, and often gestural or sensorial.[24] Attention to these forms revealed that *tension* settled in some bodies and was seen as contagious from others.[25] *Tension* even rendered the boundary between body and house, house and landscape, porous and permeable. Its onset was unpredictable, sometimes explosive, at other times barely noticeable. Listening to and embodying the various discursive and gestural genres through which *tension* was articulated became my chief mode of ethnographic inquiry.

As my skills for listening for *tension* developed, as I followed *tension* along fractured relations of kinship and care, a larger picture of such shifting inequalities and their affective and embodied registers began to emerge. Critically, *tension* is not evenly distributed across the Gaddi community, nor is it articulated in a singular rigid discursive genre, nor is it manifest in uniform symptoms. Some experience *tension* as a slow wasting of muscles, a seepage of bodily vitality. Others experience *tension* as a fraught and frantic surge of heat in the body, a skyrocketing blood pressure. These intimate and unsettling states open their bodies to the more malign forces—witches, ghosts, and demons—that still inhabit the mountains, inducing states of possession and trance. Some bodies absorb *tension* more than others. People who had roles in the pastoral livelihood that has been devalued experienced *tension* acutely. *Tension* pooled especially along the grooves of fractured intrafamily and intergenerational relations, where expectations of reciprocity, sharing, or respect from intimate others went unmet. People who experienced the direct discrimination or subtle humiliation of caste stigma were more likely to feel *tension*'s effects.

Crucially, women experienced *tension*'s ailments more than men, and women from lower castes and low-income families especially felt its pains. The question of whose body absorbed the *tension* of a family, of who was responsible for domestic distress, was a gendered one. Where men also experienced and expressed *tension*, they were able to displace this distress onto their wives, mothers, and female kin and neighbors—blaming women for causing this *tension* and oftentimes causing them to absorb its effects. Men could also parse tension's effects in more socially acceptable scripts such as alcoholism and could escape its grip through their mobility across the village and even beyond. Men who couldn't contain their *tension* were gendered as feminine. Over time, I came to realize that *tension* was an instrument of patriarchy—it generated gendered bodies by associating them with the feminine and associated devalued qualities of weakness, tempestuousness, and volatility. For this reason, I came to focus—as I do in this book—on women's stories of *tension*, finding within them both the conditions that oppressed sufferers and the means by which they pushed back against them.

Gaddi people also insist that the Western medicine that came with urban development is of no use to those experiencing *tension*. Neither are the plethora of alternative remedial practices found in the homeopathic hospitals and Tibetan medical clinics that have mushroomed across the valley. *Tension* is resistant to pills. It ignores biomedical categories of illness. Instead, it is intimately entangled with the invasive weeds that now overrun their pastures, with the clanging construction that fills their neighborhoods, with the frequent family struggles that unsettle their homes. It began to emerge that *tension* constituted an emic theory of distress that is a far cry from the formulations of psychopathology found in biomedicine or ethnopsychiatry.

This book follows this emic theory of distress—the ways in which distress is conceived of, talked about, and distributed across the community; how it is expressed in and through emplaced relationships with human, nonhuman, and more-than-human others. It does this by focusing not on the space of the clinic or the ritual healing shrine—classic sites of ethnographic inquiry in global mental health—but on intimate, domestic spaces and landscapes in which *tension* is experienced, and the relational lines of kinship and care along which *tension* runs. As such, this book is at once an account of the politico-economic and environmental shifts that this community has experienced in the past century, a cartography of care relations, and a multisensory ethnography of the intimate experiences of atmosphere and body. Through these lenses, this book tells the story of *tension* as it rolls in from the plains into the homes and bodies of those who inhabit the foothills of the Indian Himalayas. But it also tells the story of bodies everywhere absorbing the negative consequences of capitalist expansion, political marginalization, and ecological destruction. At its core is a central theoretical question that has implications far beyond this Himalayan world: Can *tension* travel?

Tension in a Global Context

Across the world, experiences of mental and bodily distress seem to plague marginalized and minoritized groups like the Gaddis. These conditions are difficult to define and even harder to treat. Those in the medical and psychological sciences have called this a "global mental health crisis" and sought to gather data on the prevalence of common mental disorders, substance abuse disorders, and severe psychiatric illness across the Global South. They produce mind-boggling statistics. Between 1990 and 2019, the global number of disability-adjusted life years due to mental disorders increased from 80.8 million to 125.3 million.[26] The economic burden associated with this burden of disease is estimated at about USD 5 trillion.[27] The disproportionate impact of such mental distress is clear. People who experience social isolation, poverty, and gendered, caste, or racial discrimination; who live in slums or informal settlements; who have migrated or been forced to flee; who live on the frontiers of climate change or experience natural disaster, are all more likely to experience mental distress. Yet, when it comes to addressing mental distress, efforts have been weak. Countries across the world fail to build effective mental health policies, and those that do consistently miss mental health targets and invest only minute percentages of their gross domestic product (GDP) in health, let alone in mental health. Where efforts have been made to address mental health issues, investment has often been concentrated in the expansion of digital well-being technologies, communications campaigns, or task-shifting efforts that don't go anywhere near the structural issues that generate distress in the first place. Perhaps such mental distress is not seen as a priority because its shapes and causes are not understood. The biomedical model of illness, which still dominates policymaking and evidence collection, fares poorly when applied to the complex clinical realities of distress and its florid and dynamic manifestations. Or maybe, more cynically, it is not really in any government's interest to address the drivers of distress, for the expansion of global capital is dependent on the ecological destruction, class inequality, and racial hierarchies of value that are the true causes of distress.

This book enters conversations in global mental health from an intensely local experience in the Gaddi villages of the Indian Himalayas. However, the kind of economic, social, and environmental change that the Gaddi community has experienced is not unfamiliar. Nor is the experience of *tension* unique to the Gaddis. Across India, stories of *tension* are not necessarily stories of poverty, scarcity, survival. The anthropological record has begun to chart the persistent somatic and mental complaints that have emerged during India's economic liberalization. As Lesley Jo Weaver writes, people express *tension* as the undercurrent of strain that comes with modern life in the present, and the uncertainty of reproducing status gains into the future.[28] For men, it manifests the difficulty of providing for their family.[29] For women, it manifests the struggle to maintain strained marriages and domestic care burdens.[30] As Weaver so skillfully notes in an urban Delhi context, the distinctive quality of *tension* is its very flexibility—the wide range of worries and concerns it can describe. While there is a word for "tension" in Hindi (*tanav*), it is rarely used, indicating the idiomatic specificity and theoretical potential of the term itself. She notes that for her urban middle-class interlocutors, *tension* stemmed primarily from modern pursuits like going to movie theaters, eating in restaurants, driving in traffic, and waiting in long lines and signaled the deterioration of the social fabric that issued from such pursuits.[31]

As for Weaver's interlocutors, *tension* for the Gaddis emerged from this thick web of status concerns—the aspirational, speculative concerns of accumulation amid the growing inequality of a cash economy. Bodies with *tension* are not scrawny or hungry; they are not riddled with the diseases of the poor (tuberculosis, polio, leprosy) nor with the diseases of the city (cholera, diphtheria, hepatitis). Instead, these bodies are fattened on diets of rice and junk food and suffer sedentary sicknesses like high blood pressure or diabetes. These minds are more concerned with how to manage house extensions, land deals, loan repayments for scooters or white goods, new business ventures, lost job contracts, good marriage matches, school fee payments, or college enrollments. *Tension* is about managing these worldly concerns as part of the struggle to maintain a footing on the precarious lower rungs of the Indian middle class. It is in this sense that the Gaddi case parallels the experience of many marginalized groups across India, and indeed across the global majority, who dwell on the frontiers of capital expansion. But existing accounts tell the story of *tension* and similar conditions from the urban slum, or busy city hospital, that is so often the setting for tales of contemporary psychosomatic distress. A far more unsettling story remains to be told of *tension* at the margins, in a place that is yet to undergo the full set of transformations that have swept through urban areas, in a place where concerns of ecological destruction frame experiences of social mobility.

THE HIMALAYAS ARE ONE such place. The Western Himalayan region has undergone rapid development since Indian economic liberalization in 1991. Deep tunnels have been carved through the heart of the mountains. Roads have been built to reach the most far-flung villages. Farms have transformed into towering hotels. The local people have been the strongest advocates for this campaign—constructing hydropower dams and hotels, shepherding tourists rather than goats through the foothills—as they aspire for inclusion in a liberalizing India. This region has also, however, been at the frontier of climate disaster. The communities of the Western Himalayas have watched as the glaciers above them melt, swelling rivers and causing catastrophic thunderstorms and floods. They have attempted to shield their animals and crops from erratic weather conditions and the blight they bring. They have accepted their previously pure water sources becoming polluted with plastic packets and the toxic waste that spills over from construction sites.

Yet, at the same time, the ecology and geography of the region have become sacralized in new ways. On one hand, the Dev Bhumi has taken on new meaning as the frontier of sacred Hindu territory. As Radhika Govindrajan writes of neighboring Uttarakhand, "The state and business investors have fuelled the explosive rise of a *dharmic* (religious) industry—a network of gurus, ashrams, yoga and wellness retreats, and temples—that claims to draw its own potency from the *shakti* (creative power) of the *Devbhumi*."[32] Claims to this land are entwined in new ways with both processes of speculative accumulation and retellings of religious history.[33] On the other hand, the intensification of thermal landscapes in the plains—including skyrocketing temperatures and toxic pollution—make the pure air of the Himalayas even

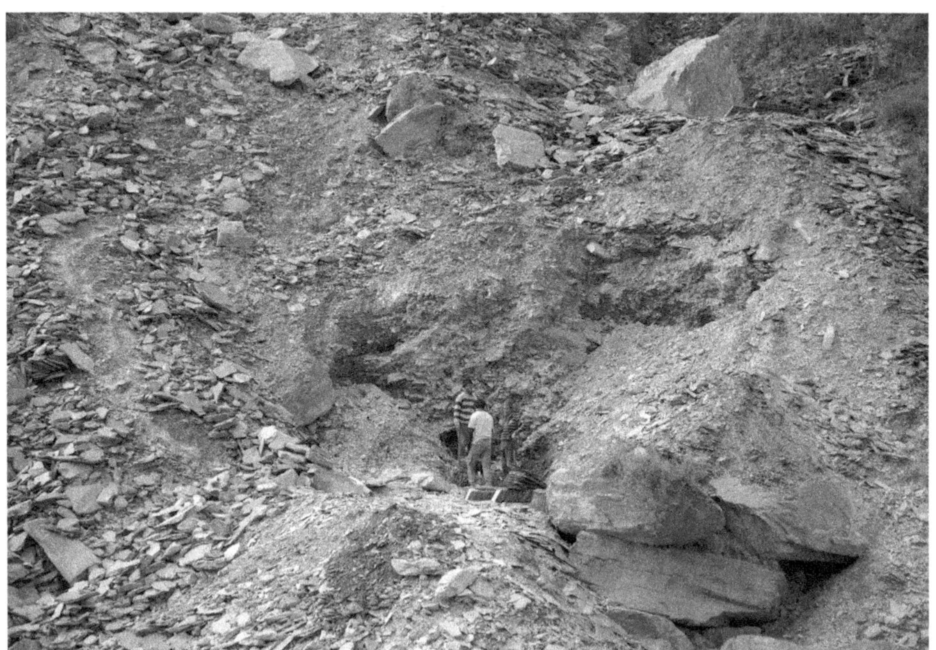

FIGURE I.3. Men work in the slate mines at the foothill of the Dhaula Dhar. Photograph by Soujanyaa Boruah, 2024.

more desirable to tourist and settler alike. Protectionist measures introduced by the state, like the enclosure of land in nature parks and closure of extractive industries like slate mining, render the landscape both the perfect victim of and the perfect solution to ecological destruction and climate disaster. The Gaddis sit in an awkward position in relation to both senses of sacred geography such that what it means to be a custodian of, or "indigenous" to, this land is in question.

The Himalayan context provides a microcosm for the study of ecological distress because the loss of majestic natural beauty that has come with development and climate change is so acute. However, it is not hard to see how this complex story might also be told for marginal groups across India's Sundarbans mangroves, Tamilian forests, or Goan coastlines. It is not hard to see how it might resonate with peoples who have experienced dispossession in Australia, the Amazon, or the Gran Chaco. The links to livelihood loss in the West Papuan jungle, the Scottish Munros, or the Tibetan Plateau might comparatively be drawn.[34] This book watches as people who held vital bonds to land and livelihood experience ambivalent affects toward the rapid change that is characteristic of the fraught present. And yet the Gaddi case offers a unique contribution to emergent conversations surrounding ecological distress, for Gaddi claims to autochthony do not mesh well with either the global discourses of Indigenous self-determination or Indian Adivasi political struggles.[35] Indeed, the Gaddi case reveals the purity politics and perversions of scale at play in the theorization of ecological distress.

On one level, this book is an account of a specific form of distress that Gaddi tribal people living in the foothills of the Indian Himalayas experience in the context of an increasingly fraught present. These people—across gender, generational, caste, class, and tribal divides—experience this present differently, expressing specific forms of *tension*. But as you read their stories—of complicated family dynamics, burdens of housework and care, aspirations for middle-class mobility, experiences of miscarriage or marital abuse—you might see yourself, your brother, your wife, or your grandmother, as I saw mine. You might feel your own head pulsing, or a sharpness at the point where your neck becomes your shoulders. On another level, therefore, this book is about how bodies and relations elsewhere hold distress. It offers *tension* as an emic theory of distress, but it also asks critically: Can *tension* travel?

Tension's Travels

Today, in English dictionaries, *tension* is defined as a feeling of worry and stress that makes it impossible to relax. But it also has a relational meaning—"a situation in which people do not trust each other, or feel unfriendly towards each other, and that may cause them to attack each other." And it has a physical meaning—"the state of being stretched tight; the extent to which something is stretched tight."[36] In each of these meanings, we see a state or condition, a bounded temporal and spatial pause, a moment between relaxation and snapping, an impasse. When people use the word *tension*, these meanings are often read into each other. The body in a state of anxiety feels its muscles constrict and stretch tight, inducing changes in blood pressure, hormones, breath, and bowels.[37] The relational state of distrust, suspicion, and jealousy is felt in the ruminating mind, in the inability to relax. The physical state of strain between structural forces, opposing tendencies pulling a rope taut, is experienced as pressure points inducing relational and bodily strain, threatening the system, a prelude to snapping. When people talk about tension, they might be referring to any one or all of these levels at the same time. Their meaning might not be wholly negative—for all systems and relations require some form of tension to move, operate, or grow.

The etymology of *tension* involves a journey across epochs of medical and social thought. Following this journey reveals that tension has always acted as a prism for gendered, racialized and classed notions of the body—used as a morally charged and biologically encoded means of differentiating or stabilizing forms of social stratification. The term can be traced to the Latin *tens* (to stretch). Its first uses are noted in sixteenth-century France, as a medical term denoting a condition of being stretched or strained. It grew in usage over the course of the seventeenth and eighteenth centuries and came to be associated with the "nerves," as a kind of nervous strain. Tension was used by the French medical nosologist Boissier de Sauvages in 1772 to describe a condition of bodily pain and social withdrawal caused by *panophobia phrontis*, also called *worry*.[38] Herein, the term was nested in the idea of the "Body as Machine"—wherein Protestant concerns of productivity converged with a doctrine of materialism that, as the cultural psychiatrist Sushrut Jadhav puts it, saw "the Body [as] a source of energy capable of transforming universal natural energy into mechanical work."[39] As Jadhav recounts, drawing on foundational historical material compiled by Anson Rabinbach, the "Body as Machine" thesis was popularized by the French physician and philosopher, who saw the body as analogous to a "watch-spring with unique self-winding qualities."[40] Within this model, tension is a hydraulic quality that both permits and prevents motion. When it does the latter, it becomes associated with fatigue, the antithesis of productivity.

In the twentieth century, physicians became interested in measuring and defining different states of such fatigue. One of the most notable of these figures was the German psychiatrist Emil Kraepelin, who sought to plot out different types of fatigue through experiments on factory workers in his laboratory. Kraepelin's experiments dovetailed with the works of psychiatrists like George Miller Beard, Jean-Martin Charcot, and Charles Féré, who sought to pinpoint the forms of fatigue that issued from nervous states coming from the brain and spinal cord.[41] In his 1909 psychiatric treatise, Kraepelin defined tension as one such state, describing the association of inner tension with anhedonia—or the inability to feel pleasure—that permeates both the body and the mind. Such a description of tension as a nervous condition of impaired energy echoes Marxist notions of alienation produced by the reduction of the body to a machine in the capitalist system. Capitalism, Karl Marx writes, "squanders human lives . . . and not only blood and flesh, but also nerve and brain."[42] However, most physicians of the time framed tension not as a condition of labor but as one of race—a hereditary condition that affected groups who were considered resistant to work.[43] The most prominent theorist of such racialized, social Darwinist notions of tension was the French psychologist and physician Pierre Janet. Janet, as recounted by Rabinbach, postulated a theory of psychological tension that involved a hierarchy of energies required for different types of activities.[44] In his model, emotions were a "variety" of fatigue in the context of a psyche that was constantly struggling between the economies of energy and fatigue.

The "Body as Machine," and its notions of fatigue, exhaustion, and nervous tension, also had influence over physicians in India, who came to modernist, industrial notions of embodiment under the yoke of British colonial rule in the nineteenth and twentieth centuries.[45] The British colonial project worked through the diffusion of regimes of embodiment that instituted hierarchies of race, substance, and sentiment. This was not a straightforward process of hegemonic dominance, as the historian David Arnold shows, but an ongoing epistemic struggle between pluralistic regimes.[46] One such epistemic struggle is articulated in the writings of David Chowry Muthu—a London-trained tuberculosis specialist who, as Bharat Venkat recounts, left his sanatorium practice in England to travel across India. In his writings, we find a vision of the body as machine—"a system of nerves, capable of both vitality and exhaustion."[47] This body is threatened by the unceasing labor of the colonial-industrial complex and the forms of urban life that go with it. The body, mind, and soul are depleted by such conditions, resulting in forms of nervousness that were not a problem of the individual but a product of colonial oppression and extraction that did not suit the embodied constitution of Indian peoples. As Venkat puts it, "What the nervous body exposed was a weakness that threatened to slide into racial degeneracy."[48] Herein we see the racialized regimes of embodiment implicit in theories of tension proposed by French physicians like Janet were overturned by their colleagues in the colonies. For Muthu, the solution to both tuberculosis and nervousness was freedom from confinement by the colonial state. Such examples help us to question whether and how *tension*, as it is used in contemporary India, might be seen as inherently decolonial—in the sense that *tension* is a term taken from colonial psychiatry and resignified in a place that has experienced the hardest edges of colonial governance, extraction, and dispossession and that experiences its most acute ongoing legacies in gender, caste, and tribal inequality and ecological destruction. We begin to feel out the ways in which tension allows us to reflect on power.

Tension has been the impetus for such reflections by another psychiatrist of colonial rule, Frantz Fanon. "The native's muscles are always tensed," Fanon writes in *The Wretched of the Earth*. "You can't say that he is terrorized, or even apprehensive. He is in fact ready at a moment's notice to exchange the role of the quarry for that of the hunter. The native is an oppressed person whose permanent dream is to become the persecutor."[49] Fanon uses muscular tension as a central metaphor to articulate how this oppression works through the body and causes distress. Specifically, tension indicates an embodiment of repressed temporality. Fanon writes, "The problem considered here is one of time. Those Negroes and white men will be disalienated who refuse to let themselves be sealed away in the materialized Tower of the Past. For many other Negroes, in other ways, disalienation will come into being through their refusal to accept the present as definitive."[50]

For Fanon, tension is the product of systems of structural oppression that petrify history and seal the present. Psychological healing and liberation exist together in moments when colonized people break with the history that is distorted by colonizers and restore an agentive sense of narrative time.[51] Interpreting Fanon's arguments, the cultural theorist Darieck Scott suggests that muscular tension speaks to both the ways in which racialized bodies hold time as distress and the ways in which they hold the potential for resistance. "The muscles, in contraction or tension, are a metaphor referring to some reservoir of resistance to the colonizer's acts of subjugation and enslavement."[52] For Scott, Fanon's reflections frame tension as a form of "power in the midst of debility" that is held in the body.

Thinking about *tension* alongside decolonial thinkers—or allowing them to "haunt" the writing of distress—helps us to understand that this state of strain, of almost snapping, is political rather than medical.[53] It is biopolitical in the Foucauldian sense that metaphors of bodily disorder are used to control and discipline intimate experience. But it is also political in the psychoanalytic sense that sensuous experiences of bodily disorder, and the bodily scripts used to describe them, are often inchoate sources of resistance—as Mark Nichter first argued in his conception of "idioms of distress."[54] In these instances, the articulation of distress both registers the postcolonial relation and opens the possibility of its refusal.

IRONICALLY, THE ENTRY OF the English term *tension* into twenty-first-century popular Indian parlance is, quite literally, about power. The term gained popularity through electrical voltage warning signs.[55] These signs, ubiquitous to urban infrastructure, warned people of "high-tension" electrical cables that were dangerous if touched. The fluid and porous metaphor of power in the built environment and in the body is repressed or transformed, however, in contemporary psychiatric and psychological uses of the term. In the psychiatric clinic, tension has come to be associated with an individualizing, mentalist diagnosis of anxiety and with wider psychosomatic conditions such as chronic fatigue disorder and myalgic encephalomyelitis.[56] Within these conditions registered in the *Diagnostic and Statistical Manual, Fifth Edition*, the Freudian psychoanalytic cleavage of body from mind prevails—where the origin of bodily symptoms is psychological, and the origin of psychological symptoms can be located in individual traumatic developmental, often libidinal, events.[57] Such Freudian "conversion" models of symptomology, João Biehl and Amy Moran-Thomas note, are both individualizing and universalizing—foreclosing the possibility of the symptom as relational, a necessary condition for an individual to establish new relations to the world or to others.[58]

Both relationality and politics are missing from the psychiatric and psychological literature on tension in South Asia, where *tension* has been used as a synonym for "stress," a biopsychosocial illness that afflicts the individual body or mind.[59] Psychiatrists suggest that *tension* presents itself as a cultural manifestation of psychological symptoms consistent with universal common mental disorders like depression and anxiety, and somatic symptoms such as dizziness, asthma, diarrhea, fever, and nonspecific aches and pains.[60] Contextually, *tension* has been associated with poverty and deprivation, a lack of education, and exposure to violence, particularly intimate partner violence.[61] However, the equation of *tension* with terms such as *stress* or pathologies such as depression or anxiety continues to obscure the way that distress is embedded in and generated through politicized networks of social relations.

This fractious genealogy shows that *tension* has already traveled across space and time. But how far might it travel still? In this book I attempt to restore the relational and political significances of tension, thus recuperating it as an analytic through which to understand the cumulative psychic and embodied costs of social, political, and economic change. I offer ethnography as a way of finding, conceptualizing, and rendering distress, a way that centers wider structural processes that shape psychic and bodily worlds, without allowing such structures to erase the nuanced experiences of those who suffer it. I examine how and why distress is bound to forms of dispossession, inequality, and social change, without reducing such forms to rigid etiologies. I do this by following one community through a set of social, political, and economic changes and tracking how distress is generated in ways that cut through dominant linear narratives of development and progress, on one hand, or moral decline and loss, on the other.

Critically, this book does not argue that *tension* can be explained by or attributed to any medical condition or particular "uniform etiology of neoliberalization or post-Fordism," as Bhrigupati Singh puts it.[62] It is not *really* depression or anxiety. It is not caused *only* by climate change. It is not *actually* a way of talking about caste or tribe or gender inequality by other means. *Tension* is all of these things and perhaps, in some cases, none of them. In this book I resist the urge to explain away *tension*, or to try to wrestle its multiple manifestations into neat categories of illness like the "cultural syndrome," or even to chart out a defined communicative purpose as part of a personal symbol or "idiom of distress."[63] Herein, I am sensitive to Arthur Kleinman's warnings about "category fallacy," where nosological categories—generated by psychiatrists or anthropologists—are reified and misleadingly applied to members of other cultures for whom they lack coherence or validity.[64] Instead, I lean into the layered, chameleonic, and ambivalent nature of distress: how people attribute it at different moments to different experiences, how it might appear acutely and then, just as quickly, ebb away. I do this by using the semiotic tools of canonical medical anthropology but deploying them outside of biomedical epistemic structures or culturalist frameworks. I locate *tension* outside of Western naturalist or modernist imaginaries that remain firmly anchored in, and perpetuate, the purification of nature from culture, body from mind. I allow the theories, imaginations, and voices of my Gaddi interlocutors to be taken seriously on their own terms—which may be slippery, unstable, and incoherent and may contain traces of multiple "patchy" ontological or cosmological orientations.[65] If these interpretations of *tension* travel, it is not coherently across bounded culturalist worlds but along unruly currents of public culture. Ethnography is an ideal tool for this kind of examination of distress, for it offers a descriptive encounter with distress in its complex relationality that is not paralleled in the positivism of the social or medical sciences.

I lean in, too, to the political potentialities held in the act of telling tension. This involved an attention to particular politics of scale—capturing the intimate experiences of pain in the everyday and connecting them to wider forms of structural change, without allowing such structural forms to eclipse the indissoluble uniqueness of such pain. As Vanessa Agard-Jones puts it, the body becomes "a site of intra-action from which we might ask new, more finely calibrated questions about how individual bodies . . . come to be, in dynamic relationship to the worlds around them."[66] At one level, this involves describing the shifting sociology of this community—the ways in which changes to political, economic, and environmental worlds were shifting forms of status and group belonging. At another, however, it involves following feminist and antiracist methods of attuning to the lower frequencies of these acts of telling—to, as Tina Campt describes, the reverberations of social life that are "not always perceptible to the human ear."[67]

Such attunement opens me to an understanding of *tension* and its articulations as a form of politics that, as Paul Gilroy notes, is "created under the very nose of the overseers," existing fugitively at "a lower frequency where it is played out, danced, acted, as well as sung and sung about."[68] To encounter *tension* is to encounter the complex choreographies by which people from the Gaddi community navigate the fraught micropolitics of everyday life, as it is cut through by the nexus of caste, class, tribal, and gendered inequalities.

Chapter Outline

This book is not a typology or taxonomy of *tension*; instead, it might be read according to the Rashomon principle. The Rashomon technique is used in screen writing to describe a story structure in which an event is portrayed in different and sometimes contradictory ways by a series of people. It is named after the 1950 Akira Kurosawa film of the same name in which the murder of a samurai and the rape of his wife are recounted from the perspective of multiple individuals who witnessed the event. Despite the proximity of the individuals to the event, their accounts are contradictory such that the film ends without a clear sense of resolution or certainty as to what has occurred. The way in which I structure the chapters in this book might be seen, similarly, as multiple perspectives on the same relationships and events that constitute the fraught present for the Gaddi people. In each chapter I hope to give a different perspective on the same set of relational struggles and social changes, thus revealing how such struggles and changes are experienced differently across this community. Each chapter offers a different generational, gendered, or caste positionality within domestic, kinship, and neighborhood relations. The embodied sensations and affects that people experience in the forthcoming accounts ought not to be read as consistent conditions or illnesses that are only experienced by subgroups of the Gaddi community but as forms of distress that are generated from particular intersectional relational conditions. As such, it is not that all elderly people experience *kamzori* (weakness) and no young people do, for example, but that *kamzori* was used by some elderly women in a particular way to articulate their complaints. As in the film *Rashomon*, this book does not intend to weigh up and side with any given perspective, or to provide a neat resolution as to what, really, *tension* is. Instead, it offers only my own ethnographic attempts to render the accounts that were shared with me.

Chapter 1 examines how Gaddi people express and experience distress relationally. It opens by introducing readers to Uncle Piouche and Aunty Karmini, the wealthy lower-caste landlords with whom I grew close during my fieldwork. It recounts how I became attuned to the forms of suspicion, envy, and jealousy that were experienced by Uncle and Aunty's family as a result of their upward social mobility, revealing how these affects were expressed through bodily complaints of *opara* (black magic). This case suggests that wider experiences of the present are deeply fraught for Gaddi people—where changes in livelihood, land tenure, and religion have rendered forms of social precedence deeply unstable and issued new forms of inequality that cut through kinship and community relations. It shows how rumors about black magic allow people to register, viscerally, the distress that underpins dominant narratives of progress in this community. However, it also shows that the question of who absorbs distress, and who is presented as its perpetrator, generates and perpetuates inequality.

We then turn to the more proximate forms of *tension*, as they speak primarily to generational divergences in experiences of social, political, economic, and environmental change. My focus in the following chapters is primarily on women's experiences of *tension*, for women absorbed distress far more acutely than men did in Gaddi households. Indeed, distress was an axis of patriarchy. In chapter 2 we meet an elderly Gaddi woman who seemed to be looking backward in time, toward an immemorial period of abundance. In the present she appears anachronistic, as she continues to tend crops and livestock without the support of her children. This state leaves her feeling *kamzori*. *Kamzori* was experienced in wasting muscles, *low BP*, insomnia, and a general sense of malnourishment and neglect that could not be addressed through biomedical care. It worked to obliquely signify the lack of respect and care older women got from younger generations, and particularly from their daughters-in-law. It was a means by which they held the burden of historical time and sought to keep it present in their households.

Women from a younger generation, in contrast, saw the present as ripe with opportunity, as they aspired toward inclusion on the lower rungs of India's Hindu middle class. But for many, the realities of economic insecurity meant that this kind of mobility was impossible to maintain, and the realities of domestic labor left them depleted. The ripe present became looping and fraught. They expressed this heightened present through *ghar ki tension* and its bodily symptoms of *high BP*, heart palpitations, and anxiety—the subject of chapter 3.

Their daughters, or Gaddi youth, sought a different kind of future. Gaddi young women sought education and employment in the cities, and marriage matches that would allow them freedom of movement and thought. However, they were also heavily surveilled by their kin, lest they overstep the careful boundaries of respectability and sexual propriety. Chapter 4 shows how young women experienced an impasse between the constraining responsibilities of the household and the expansive but diffuse opportunities of employment and education. They expressed this impasse as *future tension*—in headaches, leaking vaginal fluid, pain in their bowels, and sometimes episodes of disassociation.

The final chapter turns to the forms of distress that women experience as time is shattered or fragmented. Women who were seen as not able to manage their *tension*, who were not able to maintain norms of propriety or respectability, were labeled as *pagal* (mad). In episodes of madness, women became estranged from time and from their bodies, afflicted by acute and malign spirit possession, or involved in erratic sexual behavior. This chapter finds, within experiences of madness, forms of agency against the odds.

The conclusion of this book returns to the question, Can *tension* travel? It sketches out a vision for the anthropology of mental health that involves a commitment to charting illness and distress against the violence of abstraction. It shows how *tension* gives us the tools to unyoke a number of modernist distinctions that plague the Western psy-sciences—between the inside and the outside of the body but also between the psyche and the soma and, even more fundamentally, between the individual with desires and drives and the external social forces or even kinship relations that stand outside of them. It also shows how *tension* gives us the tools to undo formulaic stories of politico-economic or environmental transformation through a more careful attention to the ways in which people scale between their bodies and broader structural forces. As such, it shows how *tension* speaks back to biomedical models of mental illness and refines politico-economic models of social change.

I

Opara

IS DISTRESS RELATIONAL?

Sachi Dain

The power cut lasted longer than usual that night. The fog came in the early afternoon, thick, oozing through the windows and filling the rooms. At dusk it gave way to fast rain that proved too much for the village's shaky electricity supply. I was passing through the village and was forced to seek some warmth downstairs in Uncle's kitchen. Like on most winter evenings, Uncle and Aunty sat on either side of the blazing hearth, where they were boiling a large pot of water. Uncle sat on his small plastic stool with his embroidered hat tipped to the side. Aunty rocked on her haunches, turning twigs as they crackled in the fire. Uncle welcomed me and Shankar in ceremoniously.

"This is not a night to be wandering around outside the house," he warned. He turned to the pot, which was glinting in the firelight. "If the water gets

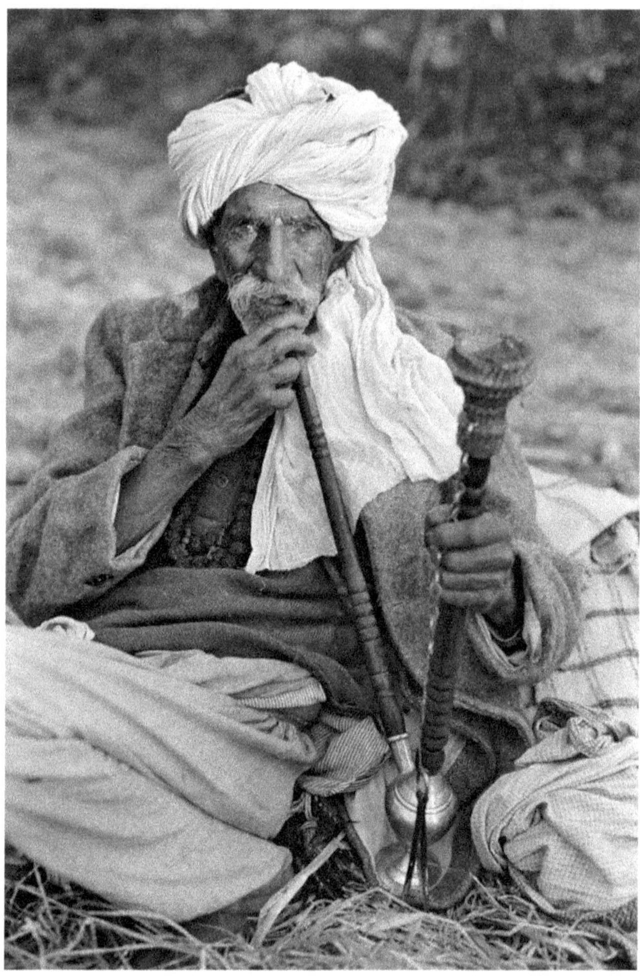

FIGURE 1.1. A Gaddi man smokes a pipe. Photograph by Tejinder Singh Randhawa, 1980.

really hot," he remarked, still facing away, "you say it is hot enough to boil a *dain* [witch] in." The stilted mood rippled.

He turned back to us, careful now to look us directly in the eyes. "The mind these days is more mischievous, for it is *kali yug*, so there are many more *dain* [female witches]. There are women here in this neighborhood who practice *opara* [black magic], *jadu tona* [witchcraft], and some men, too, are *dagi* [male witches, wizards]. I won't tell you their names because I don't want to spread rumors."

"Are they real witches," I asked, "or are there just rumors about them?"

Uncle fidgeted. "Sachi dain hai." (They are real witches.)

“Are they only in this place?” I asked.

“Sometimes they are different, sometimes more powerful, but a witch is a witch.” He spoke in Hindi, rather than Gaddi, to be sure that I would understand. “You see, in these modern times, there are more bad ideas in people’s minds than good ideas. They speak a different language to one another, so they are always communicating in these dark mantras. People these days are terrified; there is more fear now than there has ever been. I will tell you.” Uncle fixed his gaze on me, eager that I note the gravity of his words.

“They are jealous. Bad things are easy to do. People want shortcuts. They don’t care about each other anymore. They want to do things quickly these days. Before, when people were sad, they accepted that they were sad. When they were happy, they cherished that they were happy. Now this life of *sukh-dukh* [ups and downs] is not OK.”

He paused, remembering himself. “But we shouldn’t talk about these things now. This is the time when they are strong.” Soon after, the lights flickered back on, and the dark navy of the room gave way to a sobering blue.

Modern Time(s)

On the surface, the present—or “modern time,” as it was referred to, often in English—was seen as better than the past for the Gaddi people. “Life is better today,” I was told. “There is much less hard work to do.” “People are no longer poor [*garib*].” “Women are ‘coming up.’” “‘Maximum’ [most] people don’t believe in caste anymore.” These phrases were uttered to me proudly, dismissively, and were most often unsolicited. They revealed a sense of pride that almost all Gaddi people sought to convey about their position with respect to other tribal, caste, and class groups in the Himalayas and in the contemporary Indian nation-state. There is much at stake in this representation of modern time as progressive and prosperous. Qualities of caste-blindness, gender equality, and economic prosperity were at the heart of the Gaddi collective aspirational project for inclusion in an increasingly Hinduized nation, from which they have historically been excluded. Central to this project is the need to shed a persistent reputation of primitivism and backwardness that has clung to their way of life since colonial times and been coded into state classificatory categories. This reputation is echoed in the perceptions of Gaddis that prevail in the eyes of their Pahari, Punjabi, Nepali, and Tibetan neighbors. “They used to sacrifice humans,” a Pahari businessman whispered to me one day when I asked him if he does business with any of his Gaddi neighbors. “But this was replaced by goats. I once saw one Gaddi man in trance take a baby goat when it was born and bite its head off, while it was still alive, and slurp out its insides. Their practices aren't mentioned in the [Hindu] scriptures; they are made up by man. So they're not real Hindus; they came from Afghanistan and settled during the time of the Mughals, then they changed their *dharam* [moral way of life] and became Hindus."

As the twin forces of economic liberation and ethnonationalism creep up into the Dhaula Dhar foothills, becoming modern has come to involve shedding this reputation of primitivism and its associated anachronistic politics of time. Crucially, as they pursue modernity, Gaddi people have not sought to leave behind their distinctive identity, even as they give up shepherding as its cornerstone. Instead, they renegotiate the content of Gaddiness and reframe Gaddi history to prove Hindu respectability, nationalist patriotism, and economic productivity. This leads to a series of double binds—how to claim Scheduled Tribe status while also giving up agropastoralism; how to retain group endogamy as gender and sexual politics change; how to stabilize caste distinctions while adhering to democratic principles. These double binds issued multiple, often conflictual forms of modern Gaddi identity, and from these conflicts issued uncertainty, doubt, and envy, which were ultimately, I argue, expressed as *tension*.

"Modern time," Laura Bear writes, "does not become an object of inquiry; it provides the foundational questions for inquiry."[1] As Bear writes, modernity is characterized by a proliferation of (often conflictual) representations of time that thicken the experience of the present. This fraught present is pervaded with a sense of doubt—or aporia—that might be manifest in a range of moods, affects, or processes of transformation.[2] Paying attention, or becoming present to, such conflicting representations of time empirically gives us clues as to which fissures in social life generate *tension* and how political life operates through the affective production of the present. "Discussions about the contours and contents of the shared historical present are . . . always profoundly political ones," Lauren Berlant writes. "We understand nothing about impasses of the political without having an account of the production of the present."[3]

This chapter dives deeply into the fraught present as it is experienced and produced by the Gaddi people. It begins by charting out how Gaddi people are producing a shared historical present and, specifically, how this renders the very content of Gaddiness unstable. It moves on to chart the way in which I became attuned to this fraught present through struggles between kin and neighbors in the hamlet that I came to spend time in. It follows the circulation of rumors and suspicions about witchcraft and black magic as they run through this community—moored in negative affects and generating a particular mood.

It identifies a gendered split in how such a discourse of witchcraft is expressed and experienced. Where men are able to talk directly about modern time as fraught with witchcraft, women feel its negative effects viscerally, as victims of witchcraft and other afflictions. It argues that who gets to aesthetically represent modern time, and whose bodies absorb its impasses, is a question of power. In the veiled rumors and suspicions of *opara* and *jadu* that follow representations and experiences of modern time, inequalities of gender, caste, and class—outwardly denied in dominant collective narratives across the Gaddi community—are sustained and generated. Following such inequalities allows us to investigate the relationality of distress.

Recognizing Gaddiness in Past and Present

The category "Gaddi," as the category of "tribe" (*jana*), came into being as a colonial construction through efforts at enumeration of groups "living in primitive or barbarous conditions" outside of the strictures of the caste (*jati*) system.[4] Anxieties about Gaddi "primitive" behaviors and beliefs appear in the first colonial gazetteers of the mid-nineteenth century and were significantly linked to efforts at imposing taxation and governance in the Northwest frontier region. In the first and second British Land Revenue Settlement reports, colonial administrators George Carnac Barnes and James Broadwood Lyall in 1855 and 1874, respectively, were concerned with the division of land into taxable household units and the enclosure of waste (*shamlat*) land that was used by pastoralists.[5] In these first Settlement reports, the categorization of peoples in the region, the specification of their position in the caste system, and assessment of their governability through colonial ethnography were established as core instruments of governance.[6] These instruments sought to change the structure of local political authority and people's relationship to it through the specification of groups and a range of social and bureaucratic roles including patwari (land recordkeeper) and lumberdar (headman responsible for tax collection under the Raj).[7] As Stephen Christopher and Peter Phillimore trace, colonial documentation uses interchangeable labels of caste, class, and tribe to describe the Gaddi people.[8] They write:

> In the first Settlement Report of 1855, G.C. Barnes notes "Gaddi" as a general name for Khatris, Rajputs, Rathis, and Brahmins who practiced pastoralism in the hills, excluding lower caste groups. This was later

revised by Lyall in the second Settlement Report in 1874, where Gaddis were considered a "distinct nationality" composed of two classes: "first-class" Gaddis are high castes who practice commensal distancing with "second-class" Gaddis, those considered "their lower castes." [In 1919] Rose expanded this classification into four classes: Brahmins; Khatris and Rajputs (who wear *janeū*); Thakurs and Rathis (who do not); and a "menial or dependent class" that are "wrongly" included as Gaddis by outsiders but "correctly" excluded by Gaddis.[9]

While the colonial classificatory schema might have been unstable, the documentation is unified in its representation of Gaddi pastoralism as characterized by its aberrant relationship to land and land revenue systems. As is explored in chapter 2, the transhumant practices of Gaddi people meant that they posed a problem to fixed colonial regimes of property and revenue extraction. As such, Gaddis were rendered marginal and distinct against the backdrop of the new colonial property regime and its codification of space and time. In Lyall's 1874 Land Revenue Settlement report, he notes that Gaddi herders were resistant to the community management of land revenue, as it contravened their transhumant lifestyle, and the contours of grazing runs did not map onto *mauzas* (administrative districts).[10] He writes:

> The conditions of sheep-farming [in Kangra region] suit the Gaddi only. Snow and frost in the high ranges, and heavy rain and heat in the low, make it impossible to carry on sheep-farming on a tolerably large scale with success in any one part of the country. The only way is to change with the seasons, spending the winter in the forests in the low hills, retreating in the spring before the heat up the sides of the snowy range, and crossing and getting behind it to avoid the heavy rains in the summer. . . .
>
> At the end of November, or early in December, they arrive in their winter quarters in the low hills, where they remain something less than four months, By the 1st of April they have moved up into the villages on the southern slopes of the snowy range or outer Himalaya, and here they stay two months or more, gradually moving higher and higher till about the 1st June or a little later, when they cross the range and make for their summer or rainy season grounds in Chamba, Bara Bangéhal, or Lahaul. After a stay there of three or three and a half months they re-cross the outer Himalaya about the 15th September, and again stay on its southern slope from two-and-a-half to three months, working gradually down till about the 1st December, when they are ready to move off again to the low hills.[11]

The unique spatiality and temporality of Gaddi life were not, however, only material in the eyes of colonial administrators—they were also deeply concerned with the distinctiveness of their belief systems. While Gaddi people have not experienced the particular brand of colonial stigma that many Adivasi and "Criminalized" tribal groups encountered, disquiets about cannibalism, spirit possession, sexual deviance, and occult beliefs pepper the colonial archival record on the Gaddis.[12] The distinctive and marginal animistic Hinduism that Gaddis practice was also a source of concern. "The hill people are very superstitious," Barnes writes in the Settlement Report of 1855. "They firmly believe in witchcraft, and one of their most constant reproaches against our rule is that there is no punishment for witches. Every incident at all out of ordinary course, such as the death of a young man, or the cessation of milk in a buffalo is ascribed at once to supernatural causes."[13] In the eyes of administrators, these beliefs rendered Gaddi people resistant to British rule and to the grids of "rational intelligibility" that colonists sought to impose on the unruly nonagriculturalist peoples of the Himalayan frontier. These qualities locked them in an anachronistic, orientalist politics of time that prevented them from ever being truly modern or truly Hindu.[14]

"The only way in which the mazes of Hindu thought can ever be made intelligible to the Western mind," Horace Arthur Rose states in his preface to the 1919 *Glossary of the Tribes and Castes of the Punjab and North-West Frontier Province*, "will be by a scientific systemization of each phase of that thought."[15] In the glossary, Gaddi beliefs in witches—called *jogni*, *den*, *dain*, or *dogar* (wizard)—are listed alongside Hindu occult figures and festivals that take place in the Himalayas. The occult beliefs of the Himalayas stumped Rose, he admits cautiously, for they spilled out of dominant caste-Hindu characterizations. He sees his accounts of Hinduism in the Himalayas, especially in Kullu, Chamba, and surrounds, as "painfully incomplete" and feels that capturing the survival of primitive traditions requires the "flair" of "keen-witted officers."[16] In Rose's words, and in the ethnological and enumerative documentations of colonial anthropologists after him, we see in practice the simultaneous emergence of the categories of "Hindu" and "tribal"—where the latter is defined by the practice of animism or tribal religion.[17]

IF THE COLONIAL LOGICS of recognition were legal and ethnological, the postcolonial period following Indian independence in 1947 saw state recognition founded on, as Kriti Kapila puts it, the dual principles of "democracy and development."[18] Unlike elsewhere in India, caste stratification in Himachal

Pradesh is not as complex; people are largely divided into high-status castes (Rajputs and Brahmins) and low-status castes (Dom, Dalit, and Harijan).[19] For all Gaddis in Chamba, tribalness was secured in recognition of Scheduled Tribe status by the new postcolonial state in 1947. Gaddis in Kangra resided in the state of Punjab, where it was assumed that no "backward" tribes existed. As such, high-status-caste Gaddi pastoralists—Rajputs, Ranas, and Thakurs—in Kangra were understood as a caste group with distinctive customary practices. Other lower-status-caste Gaddi-speaking people (Halis, Sipis, and Dogris)—who were also part of the pastoralist economy, spoke Gaddi, and had kinship links to Chamba—were considered their own distinctive caste groups. As explored below, the latter part of the twentieth century was marked by struggles for recognition that sought to negotiate Gaddiness in relation to caste and tribe categories. Claims to both Scheduled Tribe and Scheduled Caste recognition had different objectives for caste groups within the Gaddi community that were politico-economic (to retain grazing rights, access government employment or education reservations), social (to secure group endogamy or bolster their position in the caste hierarchy), and religious (to prove Hindu respectability and shed tribal stigma). The strategies and the strategic essentialisms that Gaddi people of various castes mobilized to achieve their objectives, make up a diverse picture of what it means to be Gaddi, and to be modern in postcolonial India.

Finding the Fraught Present

I first came to recognize and become intimate with these struggles not through a careful analysis of postcolonial history but through the immersive experience of everyday life in a Gaddi village marked by the tensions of class, caste, and tribe. On arriving in Kangra, I began to spend a lot of time with Uncle Piouche and Aunty Karmini, heads of a Gaddi Hali family who lived in a village called Thera. On the brink of the slate mines, Thera is a primarily lower-caste neighborhood. It is inhabited by Gaddi Hali and Dogri families whose ancestors had crossed the Dhaula Dhar from Chamba seeking the riches of the mines. Most of these families are still employed in the mines, now illegally. The shabby, crumbling mud houses they share are a reminder of the precarity of their livelihood. However, a few took advantage of their hill-walking skills and enlisted in the Himalayan regiments of the Indian army in the 1970s and 1980s. These men, including Uncle Piouche, guarded the Indian border against Chinese "aggressors" in the snowy tundra of Sikkim and secured Indian territory against Pakistani "insurgents" in Kashmir. Today they share stories of their exploits

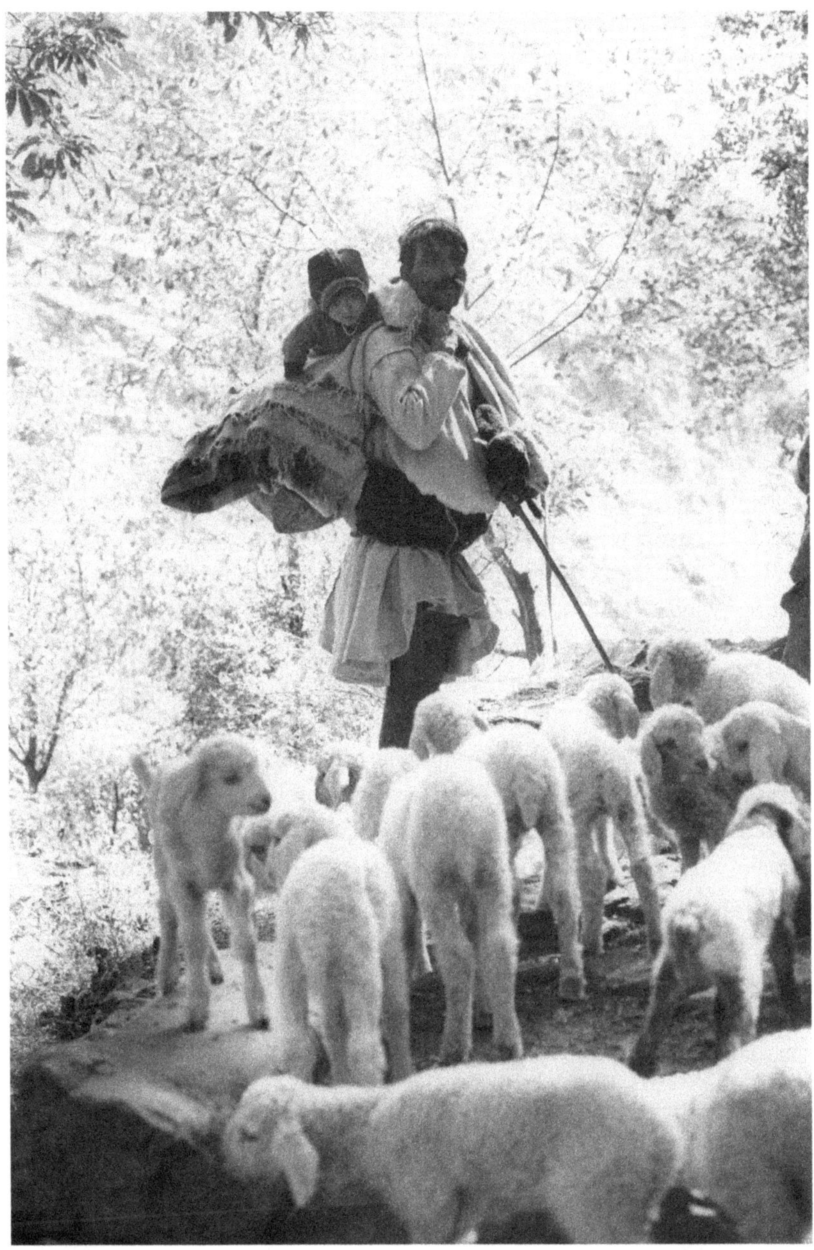

FIGURE 1.2. A Gaddi shepherd on the way to Jalsu Pass during the autumn migration south from Chamba to Kangra. An older species of sheep can be seen in the foreground, a species that Gaddi shepherds no longer herd. The shepherd is wearing a *chola* (traditional coat) and *dora* (long rope around the waist) and is carrying a bonneted child across his pack and lambs in his front pouch. Photograph by Christina Noble, 1982, part of the collection held by Noble and the British Museum.

for the nation in houses that tower over those of their neighbors and kin. The prospects of their lineages are secured by their military pension, which they often invest in sending their children to private secondary schools and colleges, and by the mushrooming taxi, trekking, and mercantile businesses they set up after leaving the service.

When I first arrived in Himachal in the weeks after Diwali, the village children's *rangolis* (designs made with colored powder) were still fading in Uncle's tiled courtyard. I was drawn to spending time with Uncle in the brightly painted walls of his compound. But Uncle's attitude seemed to echo the constant queries of my own upper-class Punjabi family from Delhi, Chandigarh, and Sydney, who were outraged at the thought of their daughter going to stay alone in some *pind* (village). "You can't trust anyone in India," my Nani had repeated imperiously to me for the hundredth time when I visited her home in the Sydney suburbs to say goodbye. While I had only smiled laconically that day, her warning nagged at me on those first nights. It didn't take long for Uncle and Aunty to share their own sentiment of suspicion with me that first real winter night.

"The mind is more mysterious these days, for it is *kali yug*."

That night Uncle's words opened a window into a lower frequency of distress that seemed to undergird his interactions with his kin and neighbors and to ripple through the wider Gaddi community. In Hindu cosmology, the *kali yug* is the fourth and last of an endlessly repeating cycle of epochs and is characterized by intensifying moral decay. It comes to stand for the present time and explains many dilemmas of everyday existence.[20] To some extent, this cyclical, sacred temporality explains Uncle's suspicions about the jealousy of others and their will to "do things quickly" without following moral precepts. However, Uncle's comments were matched by a plethora of voices that lamented the currents of fear, distress, and anxiety that shot through neighborhoods, and even families, in modern time.

The Water Tap

The water tap stood tall at the threshold of Uncle's house. As you climbed the winding road up from the Himalaya View Café, you would often see a gaggle of children milling around it, knocking each other over the head with empty bottles that their mothers had sent to be filled. The water tap had a thin, rusted pipe and a spigot that grated when it was turned, then released such a deluge of mineral-rich bore water that it invariably soaked the bottoms of your trousers. The water for the tap came from a bore high in the mountains, led down by a pipe through the slate mines, snaking past the mining villages and up over the high hillcrest of Thera, before dropping down through the pine groves to Uncle's house.

Having a water tap so close by was a luxury. In this area, water is usually provided by the district administration. This system is erratic—the water often doesn't come, the pressure wanes, the pipes leak or break down, or there is simply not enough to go around. To rectify this, Uncle Piouche had built his own water bore high up in the forestland he had purchased the use of. From this source, he was able to pipe drinkable water to the tap, into his kitchen, and to the basin outside the bathroom he used for his morning ablutions. His daughter Priya had also fashioned an elaborate chain of rubber pipes that led water into the rickety washing machine that sat on the porch, saving her from endless bucket trips for every wash.

This tap was the source of much conviviality between families—Uncle allowed his kin and neighboring families to draw water from it every evening. As the sun dipped in the valley, a long line of women would descend the mountain path to Uncle's house, each carrying an old oil drum in one hand and using the other to steady a silver urn on her head. They were often accompanied by their young children, who milled around their feet holding empty bottles of Mountain Dew or Thums Up, sometimes as big as they were. At the water tap, women exchanged snippets of gossip, inquired about sick relatives, dispersed invites to family events, and whispered rumors.

Uncle took pride in his water tap. When I asked him if he saw himself as a significant figure in the village, he cast his eyes down and pursed his lips. "I would not go into politics, but yes, I like to do social work here for my community." He used the English words for both "social work" and "community," the latter referring to his fellow Hali caste group. I first heard him use the word *community* to describe his caste when we were walking past the nearby Nag Temple, where many people were milling to pray and take *prasad* (blessed food). "Why don't you go too?" I asked, ignorantly. "That is a *puja* [ritual] for a different community," he said.

Soon after I met Uncle, the water tap stopped working. Priya's washing machine pipes lay flaccid, and the kitchen tap emitted only a dribble. Uncle set out before breakfast in his plastic boots to climb up the hills to the source. When he returned, he was fuming. He rattled on about young people tampering, sabotaging his water source. He suspected that some youth from the upper village had cut the pipe. Over the coming days, he managed to fix the cut pipe, at his own expense. However, it was not long before there was another disruption. Sandhya, Aunty Karmini's niece who lived a few houses up the mountain, had been washing her long dark hair under the water tap one morning. Somehow, when Priya dutifully went to boil water for the evening meal, the tap was broken—the spigot cleaved from the spout.

After this second incident, Uncle's patience was spent. He felt that his neighbors no longer deserved his generosity. He forbade even his kin across the road from getting water from his tap and redirected the stream so that it could only be accessed from his own home. The now-redundant water tap began to mold over at the front of his house, and in the evenings the women bowed their heads as they passed by on the way to the government tap lower down the hill.

THE WITHDRAWAL OF the water tap cemented the boundedness of Uncle's house against the gazes of his kin and neighbors. This house sat on the border between the Brahmin colony and the Hali hamlet. Its elaborate cornices stood out against the smaller mud houses that surrounded it. After the water tap incidents, Uncle Piouche and Aunty Karmini went to great lengths to separate themselves from these surrounding houses.

Uncle and his family hadn't always lived in the hamlet. In fact, the colony was the residence of Aunty Karmini's family. They had been forced to relocate when a huge landslide rocked Uncle's family's hamlet two decades before, bringing down their house with it. Some said that this area was cursed by an old widow who had lived high on the ridge. The widow lived peacefully in a small cottage in the hamlet until a developer approached her neighbors, proposing to build a communications tower. The widow protested, telling the villagers of a sacred lake that sat below the ridge—a lake that provided them with good fortune and protection. The villagers didn't listen, and the tower was swiftly erected, much to the widow's dismay. Soon the tower began to rust, the bolts that held it becoming loose. One day, the villagers heard a rumble that seemed to come from the depths of the earth. The families who lived around the tower fled to the lower villages as the ground began to give way. By the evening they were left homeless.

After the landslide Uncle procured land in the lower village and immediately knocked down the small mud house that stood on it. He replaced it with a one-story concrete building, lined by a wide front porch that wrapped around the side of the house facing toward the garden. It had four rooms—one for Uncle and Aunty, where the family's porcelain and other prized items were kept; another that had been their son Lucky's before he went to Delhi to work as an assistant in a nongovernmental organization (NGO); and a third where his youngest daughter, Priya, slept, in a big bed facing an old television, after long days of tending to the cow, the goat, the kitchen, guests, the fields, the gardens, and her own sewing piecework. I was only led into the last room once. It was a small formal room musty with disuse. Mounted on the walls were photos of Uncle in various military scenes in Sikkim, Arunachal Pradesh. He was careful to note that he and his cousin were the only ones from this community who had joined the army, leaving the others behind to work in the slate mines.

It was the stable, secure income from his military pension that had allowed Uncle and Aunty to steadily add to the compound. Like only a handful of ex-servicemen from the Gaddi community and an even smaller minority from his caste group, Uncle was not at the mercy of the arbitrary opening and closing of the slate mines for income, as were most of his kin and affines. In 2014, with his discharge money, he built a two-story concrete block adjacent to the main house, with two floors of two-room sets and a porch that looked up toward the mountains. Various foreigners occupied the upper floor and the porch, surveilled from across the courtyard by Aunty as she sat on the *manjee* (daybed) where she always spent most of the day.

The lower floor became stagnant and moldy in the monsoon season. It was rented by another Dogri couple whose children had moved to the city some time before. Nora was a plump woman with a high-pitched laugh who was employed as a domestic worker in the house of a British expat. Her husband had a distinct hunchback as a result of a lifetime of chipping rocks in the slate mines. They lived in this rented house because he had been tricked into selling his own land by a conniving brother. It brought them considerable embarrassment not to have their own place. Gaddi people who live in rented accommodation are often the subject of rumor. In their case, the embarrassment was compounded by the inconvenient fact that Nora had to work to support her husband.

In 2018 Uncle added another story above his own house, which was rented out to an Indian digital nomad. During this period construction projects had mushroomed in the area, coincident with government-mandated demonetization.[21] It was haphazardly designed and quickly built. At the border of the courtyard and the garden, he had erected a shed where a goat was tied for most of the day. Uncle had enterprising plans for this shed area. He could be found on his own porch sketching out the designs for another two-room set he would build the following winter. It would house foreign backpackers, who were coming in increasing numbers and sought rooms while they learned Tibetan at the nearby institute. He had originally been propositioned by a Delhiite passing through the village who was looking for a place to set up an Airbnb. This man had seen the mud-and-stone cowshed that stood at the far end of the garden near the bus stop and fancied it as a "traditional home stay." The man proposed to rent the land from Uncle and invest his own money in doing up the house. Uncle thought this was a good idea and promptly decided to decline the man's offer and do it himself—going into business with an outsider would be sure to make his family even more suspicious of his fortune.

Aunty Karmini's family lived close by. Her three brothers and their children lived in a one-block mud house with three separate hearths. Altogether, sixteen people occupied five dank rooms where they cared for each other's children, shared firewood and gossip. Aunty's house had five toilets: one for her family, another in the rented two-room set, another for the Dogri couple below, plus two more in the newly built upper story. In contrast, Aunty's brother built a toilet for the sixteen of them only at the end of my fieldwork trip. Before this, they would trail down to the open drain that ran along the back of their house under the cover of night.

In the biggest set of three rooms, Aunty's younger and more enterprising brother, Avinash, lived with his wife, Ruchi, and their two younger children. Over the course of my stay in Thera, the couple claimed a small piece of land by the road in front of our house and, like many in the village who did not want to make a living slate mining, proceeded to build a small shop. It consisted of two rooms. At the front was a boxy concrete room painted pink, fronted by a large blue roller door that was always tended to by Ruchi. The front room stocked daily essentials: eggs, refined oil, mustard oil, hair oil, henna, bags of rice, chocolates, chips, Amul milk, *beedis*, and matches. But such everyday items were not the source of their income. Off to the left-hand side was a room made of slate, hidden from the view of the village. Aunty's mother, Juganoo, lived with them. Like many of the Hali women, she brewed rice beer and spirits in this back room, which she served for ten rupees per glass to the slate miners who came back along the road to the lower village. This illegal practice allowed Avinash to send his sons to a private school in Khagota.

At the lower end of the mud complex, ailing Harvinder lived in the last room of the main building with its small tacked-on mud kitchen. Harvinder was Aunty's father's brother. Now in his seventies, he was tall and emaciated. He spent much of his time squatting on his porch, puffing at *beedi* after *beedi* despite his wracking cough. His wife, Loku, was a kind woman; she seemed both exhausted and resigned. After Harvinder became too sick to continue working in the slate mines, Loku took up labor in one of the hotel construction sites below the village. She would limp back from a day of carrying bricks to rest her aching knees for a while on our porch. I would ask her how she was. "*Bacca* [child], it is what it is, *tension*, always *tension*." She felt demeaned, doing the same tasks as the migrant workers from central India who hoisted their saris above their knees as they rendered and carried and cemented. Then she would shrug and continue on her way, her one remaining tooth protruding over her bottom lip.

In the moldiest room closest to the road, Aunty's elder brother, Jagjit, lived with his wife, Sonam, and five daughters whose ages ranged between ten and twenty-four. Aunty's brother was a small, quiet man who had worked in the slate mines since he was fifteen. His wife was a children's day care (*anganwadi*) helper in the nearby school. She was still young, and even though she had given birth to five daughters, her face was smooth, and her hair well kept. She always lined her eyes and accentuated her lips heavily with bright pink pencil. Sonam was a force in the village—her eyes were quick and kind, but they seemed keenly able to spot dirty laundry. She was always there, it seemed, when a fight was heard in the neighboring house or a young girl had not come home after dusk. Sonam was a mill for the rumors circulating in the hamlet. However, unlike Aunty and Uncle, she did not have a tight grip over the behavior and mobility of her daughters—supplementing her husband's piecemeal income kept her too busy.

Shifting Caste Communities

The sharp inequality between Uncle's wealth and that of his extended family speaks to a wider set of economic shifts that have cut across Gaddi families from all castes. Nevertheless, accumulation like that of Uncle's was particularly remarkable for those from lower-caste groups. Uncle's family were originally from the remote district of Chamba, over the other side of the Dhaula Dhar range. Before his grandfather crossed the high passes seeking cash employment in the slate mines, the family had dealt with animal skins from goats and sheep that higher-caste Gaddi Rajput shepherds herded through their villages. Indeed, the Halis held a particular place in the stratified caste system of the pastoral economy. Hali families dealt with animal carcasses and experienced the same casteist stigma as the leather-working Chamars of the plains. Gaddi Rajputs would work on Brahmin land for board and lodgings while passing through on the grazing route. Sipi families (another lower caste) were the wool clippers for the Gaddi shepherds and also performed ritual songs or took the role of *cela* (ritual healer).[22] The close quarters of shepherding, and prohibitions against sharing food and other substances, meant that Halis could not act as direct servants or helpers to Gaddis along the shepherding route, this role being filled by non-Gaddis.[23]

Such caste distinctions have colonial roots. Following the annexation of Punjab in 1849, the colonial administration sought to divide land into taxable units for agricultural revenue extraction. The mountainous terrain of the Dhaula Dhar meant that agricultural holdings were small and limited, and many agriculturalists engaged in pastoralism for additional income.[24] To increase revenue, colonial administrators enclosed common or *shamlat* (waste) land that was used for grazing, thus disincentivizing pastoralism. Between 1855 and 1874, they increased the area of land under cultivation in the region by 20 percent. Professions that were not primarily agricultural, like shepherding, were more difficult to tax and thus posed a problem for the colonial administration. Upper-caste Gaddis held inheritable rights to graze, secured by *pattas*, or deeds, initially granted by the Katoch Rajas under a system of patronage. These were transformed by the turn of the century into codified, permanent, and inheritable grazing rights held by individual families, recorded in the 1874 and 1919 Settlement Reports.[25] Not all families were successful in obtaining such customary rights.[26] Those who had deeds were required to pay tax (*tirni*) on each head of the flock directly to the colonial government. The Gaddis, as such, became colonial subjects through this new propertied relation to the state, as put by the colonial administrator Lyall: "The Gaddi shepherd, at any rate, who pays his grazing fees direct to the State, still holds his interest direct of the State. He is a tenant of the State within the interest which it is reserved when divesting itself of the ownership of the soil."[27]

These land-use policies disincentivized mountainous cultivation and pastoralism and pushed Gaddi herders and the lower castes down to the plains and foothills of Kangra, originally as bonded laborers (*pahgiri*) to work on the lands of Kangra Pahari Brahmin landowners. Throughout the colonial period, and even as they migrated, Gaddis continued to retain lands and kinship links in Chamba, as well as a strong connection to Gadderan, or Brahmour—the sacred seat of Gaddi life. Amid fears that the new land market would be dominated by wealthy outsiders, the Punjab Alienation of Land Act of 1900 prohibited members of castes classified as nonagricultural from buying land from agricultural castes. This promoted agriculture rather than shepherding as a more respectable profession for Gaddi upper castes, causing deeper material divisions between caste groups that had previously been less pronounced.[28] Gaddi Brahmins and Rajputs were classified as agricultural, so they were able to sell their flocks and purchase additional land without competition.[29] As such, they could establish themselves as small landowners and begin to engage in cash cropping.

Lower-caste Gaddi families like Uncle Piouche's did not have the option of selling flocks to purchase land south of the Dhaula Dhar, nor were they classified as agricultural. However, they were drawn there by new opportunities in slate mining. Slate mines were established along the foothills of the Dhaula Dhar from the 1860s. The center of the slate mining industry was the panchayat of Khaniyara. Migrants came from Punjab, Kashmir, Jammu, Mandi, and Chamba to work in the slate mines. Indeed, most Gaddi-speaking Hali, Dogri, and Sipi families I interviewed cited the economic promise of the slate mines as the reason their *purvaj* (ancestors) had migrated to Kangra. Gaddi Rajput families also noted that their ancestors would supplement their income from shepherding or agriculture with contract work in the mines. Critically, working in the slate mines precipitated a breakdown in the caste-based division of labor, as the upper tiers of mine management were not necessarily run by Brahmins. When the mines were initially established, colonial administrators noted that there was no local class to manage industry, and thus profits were not redistributed to local communities. However, in 1868 partial ownership of this mining land was transferred from the colonial administration to village landowners.[30] They paid land tax to the colonial government, while leasing the land to a British investor, Mr. Robert Barkley Shaw, who commenced mining operations in 1867 through the establishment of the Kangra Valley Slate Company. Profits were distributed among the villagers and invested by the local *panchayat* (council) into building community facilities.[31]

These hierarchies shifted with the advent of the postcolonial state in 1947, and particularly the project of integration of marginalized tribes that began in the early 1970s under the Himachal Pradesh Tenancy and Land Reform Act 1972. This further encouraged Gaddis down the valley to take up new opportunities in agriculture. It simultaneously forced any Gaddis who owned land in Chamba to hand it over to the families who farmed it, as part of a generalized trend toward the commercialization of smallholder agriculture.[32] This legislation granted nonoccupying tenants the right to 1.5 acres of irrigated land or 3 acres of nonirrigated land. Locally called Stai Bandobast (Permanent Settlement), this reform allowed 379,676 nonoccupancy tenants of all castes to become landowners. Section 118 of the act specified that only agricultural Himachalis could buy agricultural land. The definition of *agricultural* was changed from its caste-based meaning to include cultivators of all castes. This allowed lower-caste Gaddis to purchase small sections of land, breaking down feudal structures of landownership.

However, Brahmin *lambardhars* (landowners) still owned the majority of land in the region and hence maintained a high-class status. Importantly, the act somewhat mitigated material inequalities, instituted during the colonial period, between lower-caste Halis, Sipis, and Dogris and their Rajput, Thakur, and Rana neighbors. These class divisions were further broken down by the introduction of Scheduled Caste (SC) and Scheduled Tribe (ST).[33] As Kriti Kapila details, from Indian independence in 1947, Gaddis sought state recognition through ST status based on their unique shepherding livelihood, property, and kinship links in Chamba. Their campaign for recognition gained traction following the recommendations of the Mandal Commission, which contended, as Kapila writes, "that positive discrimination should be extended not only to the ritually and/or 'civilizationally' deprived sections of India, but also to what were termed 'economically backward classes.' Thus, a new category of people emerged known as the Other Backward Classes (OBCs)."[34] The neighboring Bhat Brahmins successfully campaigned for OBC status, a campaign that could have been mimicked by Gaddis. However, to seek OBC status would be to be classified as a caste rather than a tribe, and to give up on the distinctiveness of the Gaddi way of life. This was unacceptable to upper-caste Gaddis, despite the fact that most families were giving up on shepherding, for it threatened their position vis-à-vis lower-caste Gaddis. In order to cement their caste position and preserve their distinctive way of life, they sought ST status. This was awarded in 2002 to Gaddis in Kangra, but only to Gaddi Rajputs, Thakurs, and Brahmins. The upper castes use this status to exclude lower castes from tribal belonging.[35] Gaddi SCs, like Uncle, tended to join the military or to be awarded lower-ranking government positions as sanitation workers, guards, or clerks, while higher castes disproportionately took more professional positions.[36]

THE PRESENT THAT ISSUES from these shifting forms of class, caste, and tribal distinction is deeply fraught. While the ability to accumulate wealth and achieve upward class mobility is not concentrated in any particular caste, the diversification of economic roles has resulted in new inequalities of status within and between domestic networks. The question of who counts as a Gaddi is vexed, and claims to group inclusion are made based on language, landownership, historical profession, ST status, aesthetics, and cultural performance. Forms of overt caste or tribal stigma that once cut across the community have been repressed, their outward markers denied. When I asked directly about issues of caste, class, or tribal disparity among the Gaddi, answers were curtly dismissive—an old lexicon of division had been replaced with a more secular, pluralistic discourse of rights. "We are not backward," I was told. "In the past,

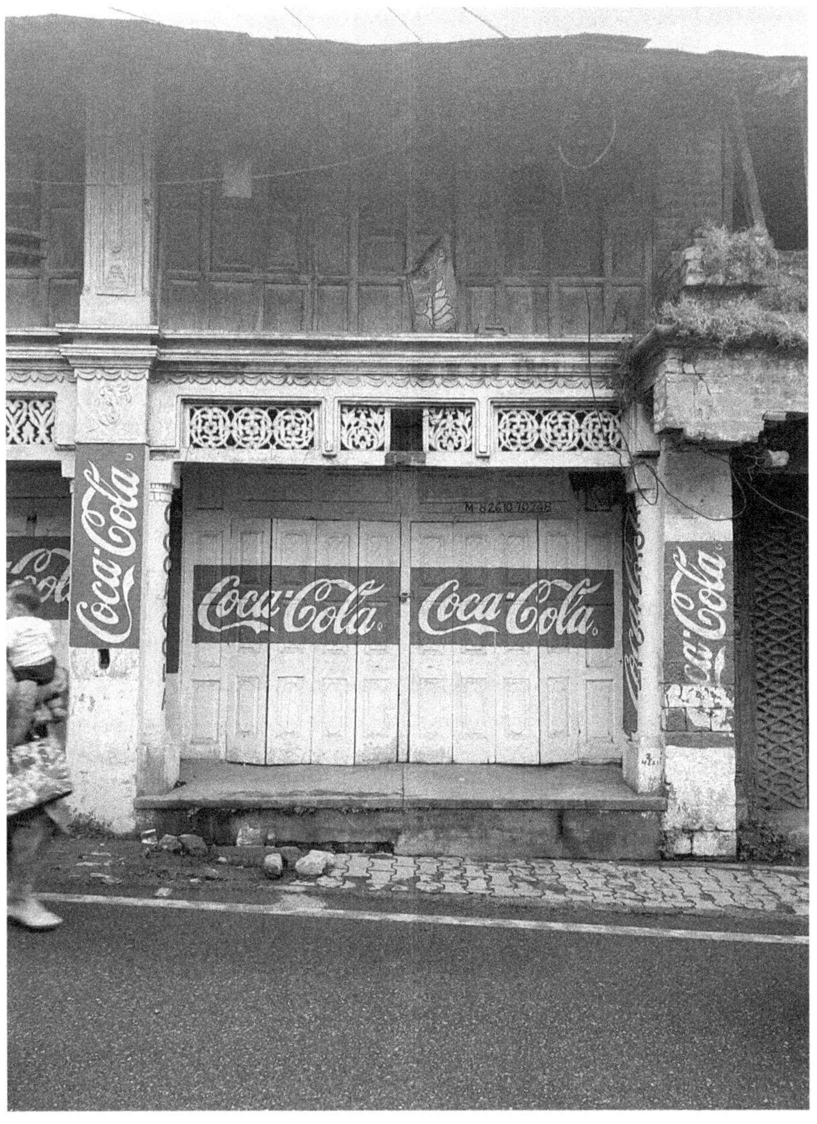

FIGURE I.3. A traditional wooden house near Dharamsala is used for advertising, adorned with a BJP flag. Photograph by Nikita Kaur Simpson, 2024.

people of lower 'community' would wear a black dot on their shoulders, we wouldn't share the same water tap. But this is no more, they have rights now." Many people across castes noted that restrictions surrounding sharing food, water, or space had relaxed significantly over recent years. For instance, men from across castes came together to drink alcohol and eat meat together at local cafés in the evenings. Lower-caste groups, in common parlance, did not refer to themselves as "dalit." Instead, as in many places in India, caste groups in Kangra were referred to as "communities" and were not strictly ordered along the lines of occupation.[37] However, the fact that caste divides were no longer discussed explicitly did not mean they weren't there, and the fact that divides were less stratified did not mean that they weren't meaningful. Instead, the stakes of integrating into a broader caste society are, and have always been, acute for Gaddi people. As Peter Phillimore observed in the 1970s, and Kriti Kapila observed in the late 1990s, the transhumant Gaddi Rajputs, Thakurs, and Ranas were always at pains to prove their parity with Bhat Brahmin or Pahari Rajput neighbors.

In the present moment, as Hindu nationalist discourse reshapes and reinscribes caste identities, these stakes are upped further such that asserting (for upper castes) or shedding (for lower castes) the markers of caste status has taken on new meanings. However, the articulation of such markers does not take overt political forms for Gaddis in Himachal Pradesh in the same way as it does in neighboring hill states like Uttarakhand. During my ethnographic fieldwork between 2017 and 2019, I did not observe significant grassroots political activism, nor did I encounter any acts of public caste violence motivated, for example, by cow protection movements. In the lead-up to and after the reelection of the BJP in 2024, participation in local grassroots and student Hindutva activism has increased. Herein, however, I am interested in the articulation of Hinduized casted subjectivities that took more subtle, embodied, and affective forms, which erupted episodically within the everyday as "moral faultlines" were crossed or renegotiated.[38] *Tension*, as I will show, issued from such experiences.

Inequalities like caste or tribal stigma take the form of veiled discourse, rumors, unsettling affects, or bodily disruption, especially when denied in public fora.[39] They become embodied and psychic. Caste, for instance, can be expressed as active or remembered humiliation, a mental and psychological injury that leaves a permanent scar on the heart, as Gopal Guru puts it.[40] It might be remembered with pain and distress, especially by younger groups who seek to repress it.[41] Or it might be articulated through forms of bodily sensation, as Murali Shanmugavelan suggests, speaking of the sentiments expressed by a leader of a Tamil Dalit community who feels that speaking with the dominant Maravar caste "is like shaking hands while holding an egg in your armpit."[42] In other words, where social life and expectations are unstable, where stigma exists but is repressed, it lingers below the level of language and consciousness, erupting in negative affects or unsettling bodily sensations. In the Gaddi case, these unsettling feelings were not just traces of repressed caste inequality but articulated a wider set of instabilities at the nexus of caste, class, and tribal relations. They were means by which forms of repressed inequality came to haunt the present, expressed as particular bodily sensations and atmospheres of suspicion that were crystallized in fears and experiences of witchcraft.

Opara, *Bhava*, and Ugly Feelings

"There is more *opara* these days than ever," Sansar, a *cela* told me one day as we sat in his courtyard awaiting a stream of visitors. They came seeking confirmation of suspicions that they were cursed with *opara*, *jadu*, or *nazar* (evil eye). *Opara* is a kind of black magic that can be performed by anyone. A spell or curse might be cast using a mantra, transmitted through a fetish, like an amulet inadvertently touched; through food, like an enchanted meal eaten ignorantly; or through bodily substances or debris, like a strand of hair plucked unnoticed. The victim would become unwell, afflicted with anxiety, insomnia, bodily pain, and sometimes possession by a malign spirit. Sansar was not the only *cela* who claimed that the incidence of malign possession and *opara* had increased in recent years—both male and female healers of a range of devotional practices agreed.[43]

Like the homes of many healers, Sansar's courtyard comes alive every Sunday when he has visitors who seek healing or wish to ask the divine about their afflictions (*deopuchna*). While some of these visitors are Gaddi men, most are Gaddi women seeking their own healing or asking for healing for their husbands or children. They harbor unsettling feelings or bodily complaints like dizziness, fainting, or *low BP*. These experiences were attributed, after lengthy consultation with the *cela*, either to *sariri* (natural) bodily concerns or to supernatural forces. Attacks of witchcraft or black magic were said to "leave the mind and the boundaries of the body weak [*kamzor*]," allowing malign forces, dark thoughts, and negative sentiments like jealousy to prevail. *Opara* was said to cause psychological ailments like insomnia, hallucinations, trance, or rumination and bodily ailments such as dizziness, unidentifiable bodily pain or ache, fever, menstrual problems, and high or low blood pressure (BP). These afflictions more commonly affected women, and particularly women at liminal stages of the life course—when they were going through puberty, getting married, or entering menopause. Often, if a woman experienced one of these symptoms, she would first go to a medical doctor to check if it was a *sariri* problem. If no such diagnosis or treatment was found, she would begin to speculate on the supernatural (*opara*) causes of such distress and consult a *cela*. As Shankar explained it to me:

> See, if you believe [in *opara*], then it might happen to you. If it does happen, and someone doesn't go to get protection or a cure, then the problem becomes *sariri* [embodied, systemic]. So they have to go to a *cela*, and the *cela* will give them something like a *dagi* [sacred thread] that gives validity to their problem or their sadness. After that, they are able to think about the problem, and slowly it becomes better. When [the problem] is more dangerous, though, this doesn't work; the *cela* has a technique, he will take the victim and perform some things, and then the victim will go into a trance, and they will tell themselves what has happened to them, [and] the Mata [goddess] will explain the problem. Slowly they will tell everything. They will then give more strict boundaries, and you have to put these boundaries in place. Like you can't put onion in your food, or you can't go to certain people's houses, or you can't eat meat or drink alcohol.

Shankar's use of the term *believe* reveals that the occult—*opara*, *jadu*, and spirit possession—is not understood or adhered to in the same way by everyone across the Gaddi community. Indeed, scholars have observed in nearby Himachali valleys that occult practices are not fixed in their communicative function or even structure, not everyone in a community or even family is committed to them in the same way, and the authenticity of both lay and specialist possession is often scrutinized.[44] Instead, interactions with *devi-devta* (gods and goddesses)—whether in everyday life or in structured ritual healing events—are meta-reflexive opportunities for the expression of doubt and skepticism about power, relationality, and change.[45] As Daniela Berti writes, "These critical attitudes towards possession need to be emphasized in order to avoid the risk of reifying and homogenizing people's discourses about possession into *one* 'indigenous' point of view which would highlight a local 'ontological perspective.'"[46]

SUCH DIVERSE SPECULATION about *opara* characterized modern times. Its prevalence was put down to the pervasiveness of "ugly feelings" in this period. "Ugly feelings," Sianne Ngai writes, "are the shameful and dysphoric traces of frustrated agency that are taken to be hallmarks of the aesthetic productions of the fully administered world of late modernity."[47] These feelings—envy, disgust, paranoia, jealousy—are inherently noncathartic, indicating social relations at an impasse. As such, they are not expressed or resolved through direct and scripted social action but circulate in diffuse forms of moral anxiety or rumor. To recall Uncle's remarks, and the stories of many other Gaddis, the present epoch is characterized by these ugly feelings, and they are particularly associated with the prevalence of witches. "You see, in these modern times, there are more bad ideas in people's minds than good ideas." "People are terrified. They are jealous."

As I spent more time in Thera, and with the Gaddi community in general, I came to realize that such ugly feelings were not necessarily attributed to particular events or occurrences. Instead, they seemed to be a mood that characterized modern time. The mood of the place was referred to using the Hindi words *mahaul* and *bhava*. The concept of *bhava* has been interpreted in Hindu and Buddhist philosophy as both an emotional state of mind or body and an existential state of being. In the former sense, Sheldon Pollock writes, "*bhava* is an emotion or mood that is less psychological" (read in the mind) "and more affective and physical" (in the relations or body), "a state that may incite emotions or may carry emotions within it."[48] *Bhava* does not exist a priori, however; it can also be cultivated through aesthetic practice to produce particular qualities, or *ras*—juices or essences experienced in the body. The evocation of collective *bhava*, Dipti Khera tells us, has been a classical preoccupation of Indian aesthetics, where artists, poets, painters, perfumers, and musicians sought to produce or capture the *bhava* or mood of a place. As such, she argues that *bhava* is not experienced only in individual bodies but might be understood as a multivalent concept for seamlessly entwining the embodied, historicized experience of a place with the aesthetics of idealized spaces and times.[49] But *bhava* might not always be positive or virtuous. In South Asia, negative moods are also cultivated collective experiences of places, linked to qualities or essences of polluting bodies, and coded through "ethnophysiologies of contagion" such as bodily illness, ritual pollution, and witchcraft.[50] In the Gaddi context, suspicions about *opara* were one of the primary means by which people spoke about, reflected on, and expressed the negative mood of the place and registered the prevalence of ugly feelings.

Importantly, witchcraft discourse ran counter to the dominant collective narrative of progress and prosperity that Gaddis across castes shared.[51] Indeed, speculations about witchcraft were never articulated as public accusations.

They were often uttered behind closed doors, in private spaces, with trusted others. As Peter Phillimore has put it, *opara* and *jadu* are marked by plasticity and indeterminacy, where the emphasis is not on the accusation but on the currency of whispers, unspoken suspicions, anxiety, and avoidance.[52] The figure of the male witch (*dagi*) and female witch (*dain*) worked to link a wider mood of uncertainty to aesthetic representations of the present. The *dain* and *dagi* were considered to harbor negative emotions or affects that countered the collective interest, such as jealousy, envy, anger, tempestuousness, sexual deviance, greed, or miserliness; their behavior was considered to run counter to collective values such as the will for wealth redistribution, generosity, and sexual propriety. In short, discourses of witchcraft worked to generate, in Nancy Munn's words, a "spatio-temporal underworld" wherein the positive or dominant narrative about modern time in this community was reversed, and the repressed affects and emotions that came with the social change in the present were aired.[53]

Here I locate my analysis of Gaddi witchcraft within a broader move in anthropology to undo its exceptionalism in the racialized preoccupations of colonial ethnologists and European anthropologists. As Peter Geschiere foundationally argued, witchcraft ought not be reified as an orientalist phantasm or a relic of primitive belief systems, but it might be seen as distinctly modern—the dark underbelly of social relations.[54] Nils Bubandt argues that witchcraft belief is not anachronistic in modern times; it exists *because* of the aporetic nature of modernity.[55] Charting the endurance of witchcraft accusations and experiences among the people of the coastal community of Buli in the Indonesian province of North Maluku, Bubandt suggests that for this community, witches, or *gua*, are simultaneously corporeally real and entirely unknowable. Hence, for Bubandt as for Himalayan scholars of the occult, witchcraft is characterized by a condition of doubt, skepticism, and critique. People's experiences of witchcraft affliction are marked by "a condition of being without a path—blocking people, in their own view . . . from maintaining corporal integrity and comfort, and from becoming truly modern."[56] Witchcraft is, for Bubandt, an aporia—an "intractable problem," "an experience that has no meaningful culmination."[57] A self-consciously naive Derridian, Bubandt finds the concept of aporia useful because it allows him to explore witchcraft's disquieting and inchoate events, without making them speak directly to larger social or political forces. We might consider discourses of Gaddi *opara* aporetic, for they articulated an instability of social relations—of caste, class, tribal, and gendered difference—that produced a pervasive sense of doubt. Without a stable sense of Gaddiness, and the structures of social distinction to contain it, social contexts become frayed, and skepticism ripples through the everyday and is felt out and expressed through anxious articulations of witchcraft.

HOWEVER, NOT ALL PEOPLE talked about, experienced, or even doubted witchcraft in the same way across the Gaddi community. Neither did they experience, or mediate, modern time in the same way.[58] There is an important split between those who *talk* generally and directly about modern time being a time of witchcraft, as having an anxious, jealous, or suspicious mood, and those who *feel* the negative effects of such an anxious, jealous, or suspicious mood as witchcraft affliction. Such sweeping statements as Uncle's, which characterized the whole epoch of modern time with this mood, were common among men. They pointed to an aesthetics of modern time that was used to express the moral decay that has come with the breakdown or instability of existing forms of livelihood and social distinction. Such a discourse of fear, anxiety, suspicion, jealousy, and distress resulted from an unnatural will to generate and accumulate wealth too quickly, to secure happiness without work or toil, or to break existing hierarchies of generational and gendered respectability.

The uncertain present was contrasted to the stability that seemed to characterize an idealized past immemorial—a time when the Gaddi community lived in harmony with the land and with each other. For some, like upper-caste Brahmin and Rajput Gaddis, what was at stake in this aesthetics of modern time was easy to explain. In the past, their prestige was secured by the caste-stratified organization of the agropastoralist livelihood, wherein they held authoritative ritual and economic positions. As the pastoral economy has broken down, and lower-caste Gaddis like Uncle have accumulated wealth through military, government, waged, and entrepreneurial employ, upper-caste authority and precedence are threatened. It is easy to imagine how this set of changes might be experienced in the mind and body as feelings of jealousy, distrust, and paranoia. However, such ugly feelings were also expressed by people like Uncle. Uncle broke away from the poverty that his kin and affines lived in to build a palatial compound, to send his son to work in a stable job in Delhi, and to marry his daughters to the sons of prestigious businessmen. And yet he was still plagued by ugly feelings.

Uncle Piouche's sweeping statements about the aesthetics of modern time worked as attempts to stabilize his own class, caste, and tribal positionality in this fluctuating landscape. His words reveal a deep ambivalence toward his newfound wealth. On one hand, we can see his pride of position, and perhaps an attitude of apathy or even disdain toward his kin and affines who make claims to his wealth. But on the other hand, perhaps he expressed guilt, understanding his social and material ascent to be at the expense of, and perhaps even threatened by the gaze of, proximate others. Uncle's speculations externalize these anxieties and displace them from any particular family member or relationship but also neutralize his own responsibilities to his kin. Articulating these aesthetics awarded him a particular agency that positioned him as a victim of the ugly feelings of others.

BY CONTRAST, WOMEN'S ARTICULATIONS of *opara* were never so direct. Indeed, women often revealed *opara* in paralinguistic forms—in sighs, deep exhalations, pauses between words. These forms communicated the presence of a malign mood—unspeakable or unspoken but nevertheless present. Picking up on this lower frequency of individual interaction required a form of "ethical listening that differ[ed] significantly from other modes of engaging with sound," as Xochitl Marsilli-Vargas puts it.[59] "Perhaps this is *opara* cast by my sister-in-law," an elderly Gaddi women muttered as I stroked her feverish forehead. "She has never supported me, even though we are both widows now." "I was OK until I went to eat at my brother-in-law's house," another woman said, shuddering as she clutched her aching stomach. "He is known to be jealous of my husband." Sometimes these articulations were just silences. Pursed lips after a question about the cause of heavy menstrual bleeding. Hunched shoulders after an episode of unexplained fainting.

Indeed, female, or feminized, bodies, which are seen as temperamental, especially at liminal stages in life, were much more likely to be affected by ugly feelings and witchcraft. When a curse of *opara* was cast, it often afflicted a whole family but was said to enter the household through the bodies of those who were most vulnerable. Hence, people from lower castes and women (particularly adolescent, newly married, pregnant, or menopausal women) were often considered vectors. Their emotions were seen as uncontrolled, and their bodies were considered hot (*garam*) and open (*khola*). Their affliction, if not controlled by ritual and bodily care, could spread across the members of a family, lineage, or neighborhood. These forms of bodily disruption and emotional instability are both moral and political—indexing the body's fraught relationship to the environment, and particularly to the house. While men might be concerned with, in E. Valentine Daniel's words, "controlling what substances cross the vulnerable thresholds of their houses" (recall Uncle's enclosure of the water tap), women feel the pain, distress, overheating, and weakness that issue from ugly feelings and the curses of witchcraft.[60]

Indeed, witchcraft rumors worked to generate intersubjective, embodied experiences of inequality. In South Asian models of health—glossed as "bio-moral" accounts—the (gendered and casted) body is made and unmade through transactions of substances, saps, and essences within its relationships, atmosphere, or environment.[61] As such, bodies are porous and permeable, and their boundaries must be shored up against incompatible substances or gazes in order to preserve health. When the body is breached, unsettling sentiments or qualities might arise from it. The body's humors of heat, coolness, and wind might shift, or it might be afflicted by malign external forces. So the question of who *feels* the negative externalities of modern time is one of inequality.

This is not to instate a binary between men as the ones who think and women as the ones who feel. Instead, it is to reveal that gendered inequality is created *through* the stigmatization of female or feminized bodies as more vulnerable to witchcraft and ugly feelings. While *opara*, *jadu*, and *tension* do not affect *only* women, they code afflicted bodies as feminized, vulnerable, and polluting. The bio-moral nature of power—the fact that social status is considered an immutable aspect of being, based on substances like blood, and determines corporeal, characterological, and psychological traits—means that people experience inequality and its forms of relational disruption in such fleshy and visceral ways.[62]

Let us return to the story of Aunty Karmini to see how this plays out.

Aunty's Pain

I had very few sustained conversations with Aunty Karmini. Mostly, she remained silent. To some extent this silence was a careful performance—a good housewife sitting quietly beside her husband, serving out his steaming *dal* and rice in a brass bowl, waiting until he had finished before beginning her own meal. But a different form of attunement elicited a deeper layer of this silence. Listening to this silence, and the whispered utterances that surrounded it, I began to piece together her story.

The summer before I met Uncle and Aunty, there was a "foreign" lady renting one of their rooms. She lived alone and was here to study *thangka* painting under one of the Tibetan lamas across the river. She employed a lady from the village to cook for her. The lady, Kamala, would come every morning for a few hours. One day after she had finished all the cooking, Kamala began to feel dizzy, and her body ached. Kamala's sister took her to the hospital, but the doctor couldn't find anything wrong. Then Uncle took her to a *cela* near

Palampur. The *cela* went into trance and told them that Kamala was afflicted by *opara* but was not the intended victim. Kamala's name was similar to Aunty's name—Karmini. Someone had cast a spell intended for Aunty, but it had instead affected Kamala.

By the time I met her, Aunty had begun to feel pain in multiple parts of her body. There was the sharp, excruciating pain of her slipped disc, which she showed me, holding the X-ray to the afternoon light. There was the dull ache in her abdomen that came to a crescendo during her menses, when the bleeding grew heavy and the blood drained from her face, forcing her to swallow pills that left a metallic slick in her mouth. Then there was the sluggish pain of her thyroid problem, which seemed to turn her blood into a thick goop. These different layers of pain had sedimented in Aunty's body, forming a hard shell that kept her away from others.

When the pain got too much, Aunty would curl up on the daybed on the front veranda and pull her scarf over her face, blocking out the midday sun. I got used to seeing her like this, clutching her abdomen, grinding her teeth. When things were good, she would tie the scarf around her head and get to work sweeping the courtyard, back stooped, neck bent. "Aunty, why are you working?!" I would yell if I saw her as I was passing the house. The next day, even sitting on the daybed would be too much for her. She would be prostrate and groaning in her room. She had no interest in the home remedies dropped off by her sisters-in-law at dusk. "She keeps to herself these days; the sickness gives her so much *tension*," Aunty's sister-in-law muttered. However, Aunty was no stranger to the range of healers that dotted the valley.

Indeed, Dharamshala, being the "place of the gods," is also a place where people come from across the globe to learn, practice, and seek out different forms of healing. As one walks through the gullies of nearby McLeod Ganj, one cannot help but cross the paths of yogis clad in saffron and monks clad in crimson; pass strings of small stores selling pink, blue, and green bottles of Tibetan medicines and Ayurvedic remedies; and read signs prescribing courses in yoga, tapping, and tai chi for the lost modern mind. The plethora of options available to villagers range from psychoanalysis to martial arts, psychiatry to yoga. Though graded by barriers of affordability and knowledge, such variety is mobilized by women as they seek help for their bodily and spiritual ailments.

Aunty didn't think her illness was *opara* at first. She began by taking traditional desi medicine from her neighbors, women who knew which herbs to collect from the high pastures and grind into sticky pastes and poultices. Their ineffectuality propelled her first to the general Outpatients Clinic at Dharamsala Zonal Hospital, then to a series of specialists at the teaching hospital in Bhandra, the military cantonment hospital in Kolanda, and then another private hospital in Kangra.

Aunty would dress in her best mustard-colored silk suit to visit these doctors. Uncle would trail behind her, his mustache neatly trimmed. There was anxious talk of an operation that they just couldn't quite afford at this moment, put off only until the next season when the monsoon had passed, so she wouldn't get infections, Uncle promised, or when the winter passed, so she wouldn't get a cold. In the meantime, there were visits to the Tibetan hospital for needling, to the Ayurvedic hospital for bitter brown balls, and to the homeopathic clinic for massage.

Finally, when Uncle was truly fed up, he took Aunty to a *cela* in the next town. Their suspicions were confirmed. The spell that had afflicted Kamala had now been cast on Aunty. The cause of her illness was *opara*. "This has all happened because I am doing better than the others," Uncle said gravely, as he recounted the story to me.

I WATCHED AS UNCLE attended to Aunty's pain and distress. It gripped him, making his brow furrow and his shoulders hunch. When I greeted him as he brushed his teeth in the courtyard, I always knew from his face if she had had a good night or not. Uncle and Aunty did not ever accuse anyone of casting the spell of *opara*. They did not name any particular neighbor, and they certainly didn't name any of their kin. However, as they became more convinced that Aunty's experiences were caused by *opara*, they withdrew further from those they were previously close to. Uncle prohibited the village children from coming to play in the courtyard. In the first instance, *opara* allowed Uncle and Aunty to cut their networks, enclosing their family from their wider obligations. It helped them to make sense of their ambivalent position with respect to kin, caste, and community.[63]

In expressing these sensations as *opara*, people rendered visible the pain caused by these corrosive forms of inequality and sought protection from the negative emotions that drove them. However, acts of telling also worked to articulate the ambivalence of their position. In the case of those who were prosperous, *opara* served to mark the erosion of relational bonds that was necessary for their upward social mobility, and the malign power of envy that could cause their advantage to crumble at any moment. In the case of others who were less prosperous, *opara* marked the inequity of economic opportunity, and the humiliation and frustration it caused.

Yet *opara* was not experienced in the same way by Uncle, as a man, and Aunty, his wife. For Uncle, seeing his wife, and himself by extension, as a victim of *opara* allowed him to externalize his experiences of emotional instability and affective disorientation. He did so through a collective narrative of modern time as a period of moral decay. This collective narrative framed his specific experiences of relational tension with neighbors and kin and worked to justify the consolidation of his wealth.

For Aunty, naming herself as a victim of *opara* was not quite so functional. On one hand, for Aunty and other Gaddi women I encountered, the act of telling pain or expressing distress created the conditions for a kind of recognition that was otherwise denied, and elicited care from those around them that was often lacking. This was not the general aesthetics of modern time that was enjoyed by Uncle and other men. Instead, it was the slowing down of time that came with the visceral certainty of pain, the pause in the rhythms of social life and work, that was fortifying.

But on the other hand, the act of telling pain or distress began a long chain of speculation on the part of others—husbands, kin, affines, and even me—that destabilized and overwrote the voice of the sufferer. Women, feminized bodies, and people from lower castes or classes who experienced witchcraft were considered polluting and potentially dangerous, such that speculations about witchcraft overshadowed the experience of pain itself. Hence, *opara* neither provided relief to the sufferer nor necessarily improved their position. Indeed, while *opara* allowed some people to recast their experiences through an aesthetics of modern time, it also worked to truncate the agency of the sufferer, to eclipse their pain, and to encompass it within existing structures of an authority that was often patriarchal.

Aunty's distress was a pulse that waxed and waned, radiating outward from her body. Her pain worked to pull others' bodies into relation with it. And yet the speculations that she, Uncle, and others made about her pain, the way in which it was attributed to *opara*, caused her to be seen as polluting, a potential source of malign affliction. Aunty's body came to internalize the impasses of relationships in the village, with kin and neighbors, through whisper and rumor. She was thereby stigmatized, withdrawing herself from these relations, her pain causing others to withdraw from her. She would come to be blamed for inviting these malign forces into the household of her extended network, for she was not the only one in her family to be afflicted by distress that was attributed to *opara*. We will continue with her story, and that of her kin, and come to hear how the family held and worked through this ambivalence. But for now, let us close with a foundational reflection on the relationality of distress in modern time.

Attention to Pain

This chapter has begun to chart out why the present is so fraught for Gaddi people as they struggle to renegotiate a nexus of class, caste, and tribal relations. It has attempted to bring into view the unstable forms of relationality that characterize this present. Such unstable forms of relationality issue ugly feelings that amount to a general mood, or *bhava*, of uncertainty that characterizes modern time. This mood is codified in discourses of witchcraft—*opara* and *jadu*. It is possible for some, namely, men, to articulate such witchcraft anxieties as a general aesthetics of time. However, for others, and particularly women or those with feminized bodies, witchcraft anxieties are felt viscerally as vulnerability, stigma, and ultimately pain. This book, in general, is interested in examining and attending to this pain as it is experienced and expressed by different women, as a result of different political, economic, and relational struggles.

In her classic book *The Body in Pain*, Elaine Scarry writes that the most fundamental thing about pain is that it is unknowable to the other: "When one hears about another person's physical pain, the events happening within the interior of that person's body seem to have the remote character of some deep subterranean fact, belonging to an invisible geography."[64] While the sensations of pain may be fundamentally unknowable, they issue a particular relation between the sufferer and the other—where the one experiencing pain has an immutable certainty about that fact, and the one witnessing or speaking for that pain has a deep form of doubt. "Thus, pain comes into our midst as at once that which cannot be denied and that which cannot be confirmed," Scarry writes.[65]

While the pain that Gaddi women experienced was not specifically located or purely physical, as in Scarry's writings, I realized that her thesis works both ways in relation to their experiences. When the broader experience of time is uncertain, when livelihoods and social expectations are in flux, as in the Gaddi case, then this uncertainty is expressed and experienced as forms of uncanny affliction. However, the distribution of these afflictions across the community is not equal, just as the experience of time is not the same. Some have the agency to speak directly about such experiences of uncertainty. They often do so through aesthetic representations of modern or present time. Others, however, are not able to speak directly to the forms of uncertainty and vulnerability that they experience.

Uncertainty, and the ugly feelings that come with it, settles in the bodies considered to be the most socially weak, vulnerable, polluting, or transgressive. When sufferers articulate or express pain or distress—most often indirectly, in a groan, a low hum, a scream—people are propelled into each other, forcing action, often causing time to stop or proximate relationships to shift. Such articulations of pain are made sense of through diverse semiotic forms—metaphors of heat or pressure, behavior around food or things, or the idea of supernatural beings inhabiting the body. While the semiotic media that frame such pain and distress are often deeply aporetic, these forms, like *opara*, turn the visceral, personal experience into shared symbolic forms. These work to make meaning from pain and distress and to mediate time in subtler, more oblique ways. The relief offered by such an act of telling is fleeting, but a caesura in the temporal rhythms of social life.

The question of who can make what kind of meaning out of distress, through which semiotic media, is a question of power. As such, acts of telling distress provide a form of inchoate and fleeting agency, but acts of retelling, speculating, and controlling distress often entrench existing relations of power. Here we see how attention to pain and distress, to both semiotic framings and the lower frequencies through which pain is expressed, becomes a blueprint for thinking about both the interconnectedness and inequality of people and the ways in which opacity, doubt, and ambivalence sit at the heart of such relationships. It throws into relief particular relations of power, in the words of Laurie Denyer Willis, "how bodies are never just mere vessels of the self, beings to be impinged upon by governing forces, but alight and connect as intimate projects of connection and power."[66]

2

Kamzori

HOW DOES THE DISTRESSED BODY HOLD TIME?

Nakaro Devi

Nakaro was working when I first met her. She was methodically cutting the vegetables that she had foraged in the foothills that morning, using a hooked knife positioned at her feet. The only sound was the fast click of the blade cutting mustard greens, then radish tops, then watercress. Her knees were folded around her ears in the way that only the supple elderly sit, bodies gnarled like willow trees after years of hard work in the fields. Her daughters' bodies didn't look like that. They were softer, rounded, padded, and preened.

It was impossible to tell if Nakaro was in her fifties or her eighties. Her skin sank in deep cavities below her cheekbones, regal and haggard. Her nose was hooked and pierced on both sides by the rings that marked her as a married woman. Her thin frame would still carry extraordinary weight. Rod straight, she could balance piles of grass on her head. She wore her hair in a thin plait at the base of her neck and often kept her head covered by a scarf. She didn't wear this scarf in the provocatively demure way of the younger generation of housewives but tied it practically around her head, keeping it out of the way as she worked.

Nakaro seemed to always be working. She rose early to milk the cow and take it to pasture; she attended to breakfast for her sons, then walked over to the riverbank to feed the horses. After lunch, she would go to the old mud house to sow, weed, or harvest until dusk, returning wearied by the sun. Such a regimen had sedimented in her body. She would frequently complain of weakness, fatigue, muscle wastage, and body aches. "I am *kamzor* [weak] now," she would mutter, absently. She was unable to engage with the world around her, as if she was lost in translation.

It was during her son's wedding that I really came to understand the affliction that Nakaro suffered. As Nakaro's nephew, my research companion Shankar was called frequently to her house to carry out errands. These increased in volume when the wedding was announced, which meant I, too, began to spend more and more time in Nakaro's house. Nakaro's son, Raman, had finally been matched with a girl from Baijnath, a town some three hours from their own, past Palampur. The girl, like Nakaro's family, was from the Rajput caste, but her father was a wealthy construction contractor. Nakaro's own family had not reaped the benefits of the increasingly developmentalist Kangra economy. Her husband, Arjun, still held a small flock of sheep and goats even as Raman had found a sought-after government job. Arjun, however, was renowned as a man of prestige and humor across the Gaddi community. He commanded a respect that was connected to the place and the animals that fed on it. Both because he wanted to impress the bride's upper-class father and because he loved a drink and a dance himself, Arjun would not miss an opportunity to host a grand wedding for his eldest son. He had already taken out a sizable loan to build and decorate a new concrete house for the couple.

Nakaro was notably less interested in the wedding preparations, or in impressing her prospective in-laws. When we visited the new house each day—dropping off poles for a marquee, peeling garlic for the food preparations, chopping wood for the fire—I found her milling about the kitchen or trampling across the garden, always beyond the fray of visiting relatives. "My mother just cares about her cow and keeping the horses fed," whispered Nandini, Nakaro's younger daughter, as she caught me watching her mother leading one of the horses down to the stream to drink. Even in this auspicious wedding time, Nakaro seemed interested only in making simple roti or sweeping the unused mud house. Her remoteness from the festivities became even more apparent when the wedding festivities started. In the nights leading up to a Gaddi wedding, the groom's female relatives congregate in the wedding house, bringing gifts—Old Stag whiskey bottles, thick polyester blankets from Dharamsala market, oily packages of fried pooris. To the beat of a drum, they sing traditional wedding songs long into the night. The songs tell the story of the marriage of Lord Shiva, or Dhundu, to his wife, Gorji, or Parvati. The wedding itself mimics Dhundu's attempts to escape the marriage, to run away from his responsibilities as a householder, in search of the divinity of the ascetic life. The women who surround the groom have a mythical role in stopping this escape—in the days leading up to the wedding, their songs prepare the groom for the mysteries of marriage. On the day of the marriage, when the groom tries to escape, they rush in, shouting and laughing, grasping him around the waist and hauling him back to his bride and her worldly concerns.[1] While normally the mother of the groom leads such celebrations, Nakaro remained on the fringes night after night—until the last one.

On that last night, the house was heaving with the bodies of women—aunts, cousins, sisters-in-law—who had all come to tease and jibe Raman before the wedding began. After they ate a heavy meal of rice and vegetable curry, they began to congregate in the formal sitting room of the new concrete house. With their legs tucked under them on matted floor and their laps covered by thick blankets, they began to sing. The singing was led by one of Raman's aunts, a plump woman with a full voice, who directed her daughter to play the drum beside her. As more women joined in, the sound swelled, and the bodies in the room began to sway along with it. I noticed that Nakaro had come to sit in the far corner, her scarf pulled low over her eyes, rocking to the beat of the drum.

I was looking away from her, distracted by the music, singing myself, until I heard a scream. The shrill sound pierced the room and became entangled with the voices of the women, who seemed to sing more loudly in response to it. I searched for its source. Nakaro's thin frame raised itself from the floor like a puppet on strings. She threw her arms over her head, her wrists twisting and her knees buckling as she began to pulse back and forth, spinning and tripping over the bodies of the singing women. The scream petered into a melodic muttering. "The Mata is coming." The Mata is coming. The Mata is coming. The Mata, or divine goddess, filled her body. "Take me, Mata, let me go." Her scarf slipped from her head, revealing her bare scalp underneath, the tendrils of her remaining hair coming loose from the thin plait. She addressed her son, in a low whisper now. His face drained of color, and he ran from the room. She began to run back and forth, thudding against the walls. The women scrambled

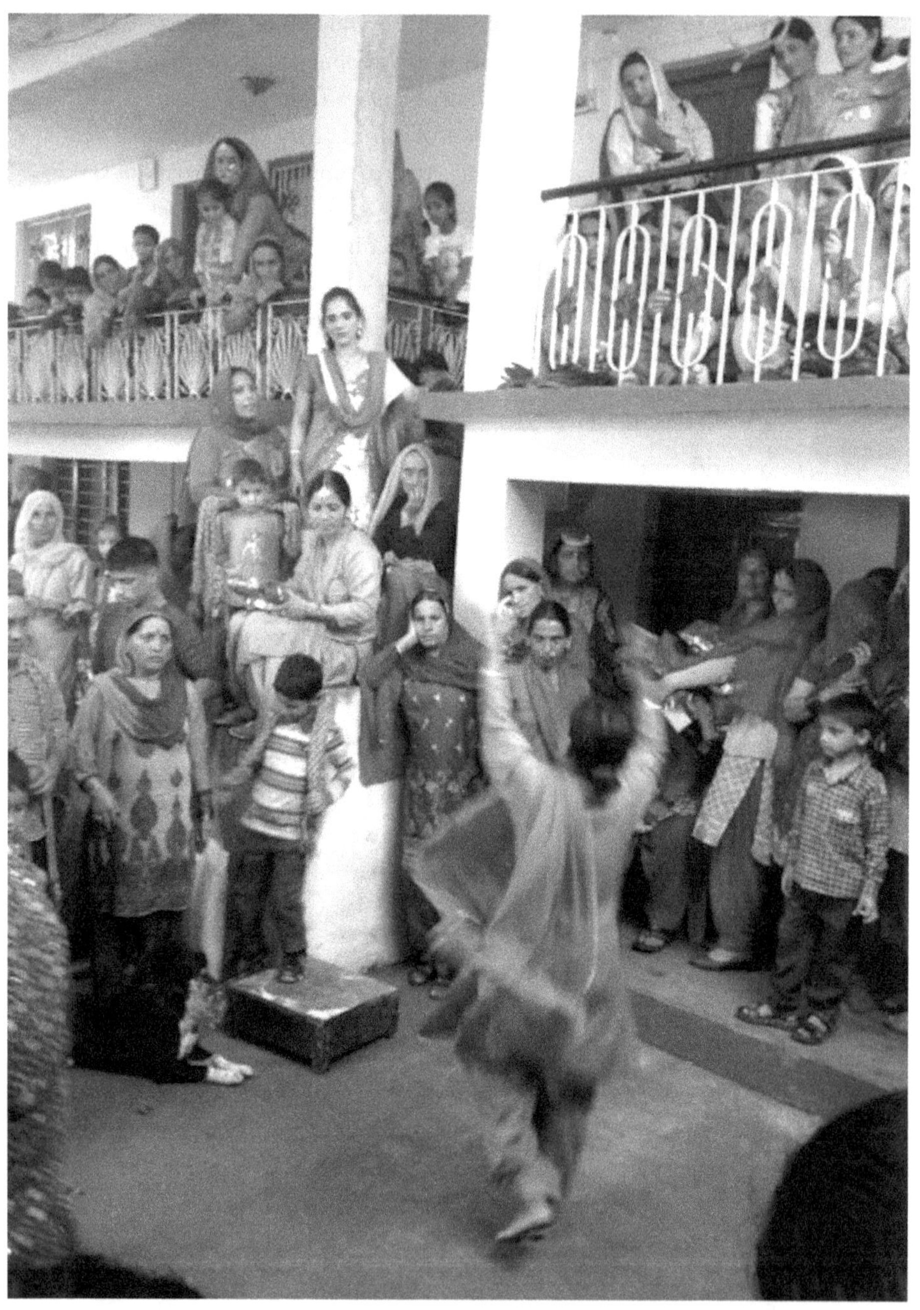

FIGURE 2.1. A Gaddi woman in a trance at a wedding. Photograph by Nikita Kaur Simpson, 2014.

to make way for her. Abruptly, she stopped in a spot in the middle of the room and began to spin and flap her arms. The women did not seem alarmed. They pulled their own scarves lower over their heads and bowed before her. A divine presence had entered the room. Nakaro seemed to ebb out of the trance and collapsed on the floor, surrounded by bowed heads. She breathed in gulps of air, and her eyes twitched open. As her possession abated, the women's voices strengthened to fill its place, and the music began again in earnest. But then she snapped back up and rose, spinning again, her chest vibrating. Her son rushed back into the room, clutching a burning stick of incense and a glass of water. "The Mata is here," he said. Her trance was long. When the Mata finally left her, she curled up on the floor under one of the blankets, pulled it over her head, and went to sleep. I watched her twitch as the heady scent of sandalwood coiled around her.

"That often happens to my mother," Nandini told me the following day. Her older sister, Sarla, agreed. "My mother [has] suffered a lot," Sarla explained. "We all [have] suffered. It was my mother who cared for us. She used to take us up to the shepherding hut, strapped to her back. Now she is tired, she can't really do anything, she can't make decisions anymore, and she is *kamzor*. We always have to tell her, do this, go there, do that. She is actually very disturbed. She has suffered a lot at the hands of this family."

In these first encounters with Nakaro during her son's wedding, I came close to the poles of her bodily affliction. On one hand, in *kamzori*, she experienced a loss of vitality. On the other, in moments of frenzied possession by the Mata, her body was filled with the divine vitality of the goddess. I was struck by the fact that these poles of experience might be held in the frail body of one woman.

THE TERM *KAMZORI*, IN Hindi, Urdu, Punjabi, and other South Asian languages, is used to describe the loss of physical and mental vitality and the depletion of bodily substance.[2] Anthropologists, particularly in South Asia, often see such bodily weakness as an expected part of the aging process.[3] As a person enters the last stage of their life and nears death, they withdraw from productive work and become more marginal in household work. The weakening of the body parallels the weakening of their attachment to kin and the natural world. This process of aging is difficult but desirable, Sarah Lamb writes, with reference to elderly Bengali women. "Denigrating flesh" is seen as a means by which the elderly signify their need for more care and withdraw from household labor.[4] Women who are successful in this process take on spiritual strength, shedding gendered markers of temperamentality, which allows them to take on new forms of masculine or ascetic authority.[5]

Some Gaddi women felt their bodies becoming *kamzor* as they neared the end of their lives. They saw *kamzori* as part of a bodily "self-cooling" process—where they avoided heating foods like meat, garlic, and onions; began to wear simpler clothes; and abstained from sexual activity or the expression of overt emotion. For too many, however, *kamzori* appeared prematurely and painfully. It occurred in moments of distress and exhaustion when they felt that they were not adequately cared for by their children or daughters-in-law, when they were not able to rest or withdraw from work. For these women, *kamzori* was an ebb, a slow, low frequency that joined the body, house, and landscape in a state of depletion. They described *kamzori* as a loss of *shakti* (or libidinal life force) and *takat* (physical strength) that led to feelings of exhaustion and lethargy. Bodily, it was felt in wasting muscles, weight loss, joint pain, back pain, *low BP* (low blood pressure), disrupted digestion, stomach pain, and appetite loss. It marred the mind with insomnia, hallucinations, and confusion. *Kamzori* could leave the boundaries of the body permeable and render one vulnerable to attacks of *opara*. Women who experienced *kamzori* argued that it would not be alleviated with biomedical care. Instead, it rendered the body resistant to medication and nourishment. As such, the illness was somewhat of a mystery to medical doctors in the Dharamsala Zonal Hospital and was often explained as a psychosomatic complaint.

Kamzori, in this acute sense, was also often accompanied by erratic episodes of spirit possession, wherein the body was filled with the spirit of a fearsome, divine goddess. This often happened in public events such as a marriage or ritual, where the woman's body would move frenetically, running, jumping, dancing, shouting, unaware of its surroundings, in pulsating movements. When the state of possession abated, the woman would return to her state of exhaustion, often not remembering or acknowledging what had just happened. This kind of possession was not considered problematic. Instead, it afforded the woman a form of awesome prestige, albeit for a moment.

"WHAT IS THE BODY?" Gilles Deleuze asks in his essay "Active and Reactive." "We do not define it by saying that it is a field of forces or a nutritive medium in which a plurality of forces quarrel. For in fact there is no 'medium,' no field of forces or battle. And there is no quantity of reality, for all reality is already a quantity of force. There are nothing but quantities of force 'in a relation of tension' between one another."[6]

For Nakaro and other women who experienced premature *kamzori*, these two forces—weakness and divine strength—existed simultaneously and in tension with each other, constituting their experience of their own bodies in relation to the intimate others around them. Considering Deleuze's writings, Bhrigupati Singh suggests that anthropologists have a unique role to play in charting, or even measuring, the "waxing and waning" of these forces across the lives of their interlocutors.[7] When Singh returned to his field site, a village in Rajasthan, after a long absence, he was struck by changes that had occurred in his interlocutors' lives. Asking the simple question "How are you?" elicited measurements of both individual life events and wider shifts in kinship networks, livelihood conditions, and environmental prosperity. "What to do sir, some of it is *samay* (the burden of 'time'—referring to unnamed events specific to his life), some of it is *zamana* (the times we live in)," one of his interlocutors philosophized, using a familiar adage.[8]

How do bodies hold the burden of time? How do they adapt to or resist the times? These questions are shared to some extent by any community that has undergone a change in livelihood. They are particularly prescient for Indigenous and marginalized groups, like the Gaddi, for whom this change involves an existential rupture. This chapter dwells on these questions through a particular attention to the waxing and waning of one life. This life, Nakaro's life, may not be considered normal or even representative of Gaddi women's experiences, but neither is it esoteric or even marginal. Instead, it speaks to a wider waxing and waning of collective vitality—what Gaddi people referred to as *dharam*, or the moral way of life that was generated through connection to place, practice of the unique pastoral livelihood, spirituality, and kinwork. The notion of *dharam* scaled between the landscape, the household, and the body. It bound together concerns of health, well-being, gendered and casteist respectability, domestic organization, and connection to landscape and animals. It was achieved through particular forms of *kaam* (work, labor) that were part of the shepherding economy and involved the exertion of life force on the world.[9] The moral decay that came with the breakdown of *dharam* and the loss of vital *kaam* was felt especially in the breakdown of generational relations, the cleavage of the elderly from the young. Elderly people were most concerned with a loss of self-sufficiency that came with the breakdown of *dharam*. They lamented younger generations' dependency on the state and market, and their lack of respect or care for practices of traditional work. While some were able to adapt to the times, many elderly people felt out of place or temporally disoriented in the present. Their bodies held the burden of a Gaddi history that they felt was almost lost. However, holding on to history at the level of the body was

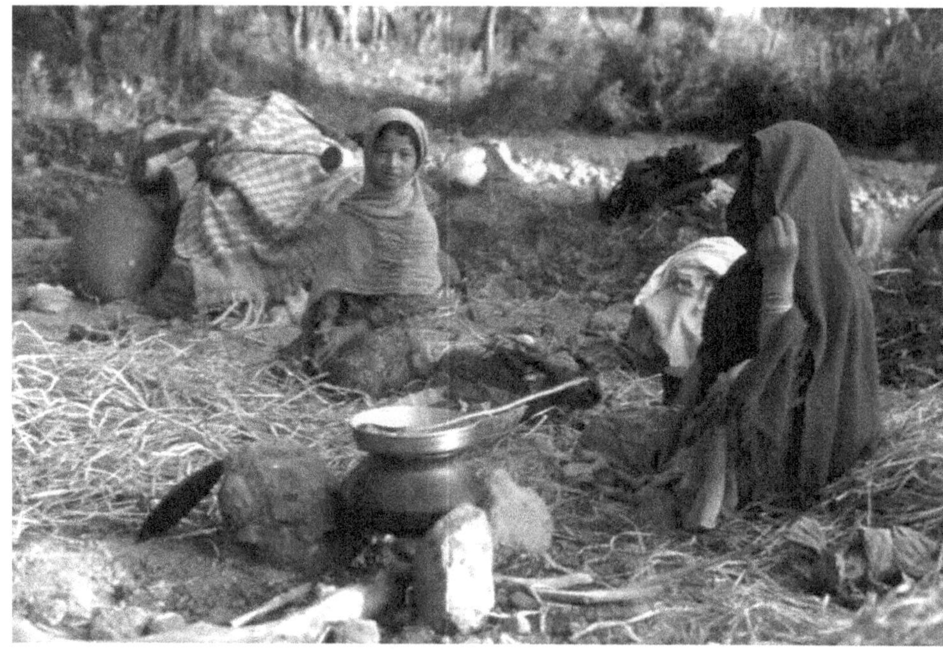

FIGURE 2.2. A Gaddi woman and her daughter make camp in the Shivalik hills. The woman practices *ghoonghat*—hiding her face from male onlookers with her scarf. Photograph by Tejinder Singh Randhawa, 1980.

also a means by which they resisted such change and sought a different future for their community. As we will come to see, Nakaro's experiences of *kamzori* and possession speak to this wider waxing and waning of Gaddi life over time.

A Lived History

Nakaro's family was from a village in the next valley. She had grown up in a shepherding family—her father and then her brothers had herded their flocks from their house in Chamba across the Dhaula Dhar to their shepherding hut in the Kangra hills, then through the ancient Shivalik hills into the Punjab plains. The trials that faced Nakaro's ancestors (*purvaj*) mirror the wider challenges faced by the Gaddi community as their livelihood shifted. Nakaro's position in this story is critical, in terms of both her generation and her gender. She sits on a precipice of time between one way of life and another, one form of Gaddi femininity and another. Nakaro's generation grew up in a world where the shepherding economy structured intimate, spiritual, and economic life, but they grow old in another world, where such a livelihood has become obsolete. For women, this experience is particularly acute—where shifts in the shape of respectable Gaddi femininity have run parallel to livelihood change. I only began to truly understand Nakaro's life experience when I looked back into the archive and began to trace the British colonial legacy through to the present. I began to see the way in which colonial grids of legibility—instituted through the categorization of people, the enclosure and taxation of land, the standardization of marriage and inheritance practices—shaped generational change in this community. I pieced together this story with fragments of oral history provided by elderly people, who were only too keen to talk about their past. Let us take a moment now to trace this history.

Upper-caste Gaddi flock owners, Nakaro's ancestors included, were granted inheritable land access rights by the Katoch Rajput Rajas of Kangra and Chamba prior to the annexation of Punjab by the British Raj in 1849. Gaddi herders were granted by the rajas the hereditary—but not inalienable—right to graze, which was renewed through skilled engagement with king and court. There was no distinction among public, communal (*shamlat*), and private land.[10] The head of the flock (*mahlundi*) was he who held this claim (*warisi*) from the raja. Nominally, it was he who dealt with the tax arrangements with the raja and the local village community—entitling him to use the *ban* (summer pastures) and *dhar* (alpine pastures).

In his 1874 Land Revenue Settlement, J. B. Lyall recounts this historical relationship:

> In former days there were more woods and fewer flocks. An enterprising shepherd came across an unoccupied tract: he hung about the Rajah's court till he got access, when he presented a "nazar" or offering, and made his application. If his "nazar" was accepted, he got a *pattah* authorising him to graze sheep in the place applied for. Armed with this *pattah*, he set about forming a company of shepherds to join him in grazing the new "ban." Next year, when the time came round to descend into the low country, the members of the company brought together their contingents of sheep and goats, and the flock was formed, The holder of the *pattah* directed the course of the flock, and acted as spokesman and negotiator in case of quarrels or dealings with the people along the line of march.[11]

This relationship of patronage is represented by colonial administrators as one of hierarchy, where rajas controlled their tribal subjects through land grants and tributes paid for crossing certain villages. Lyall refers to such taxation as a form of "*suzeraineté* over the race."[12] However, both scholarship and Gaddi oral histories suggest that this relationship might be more accurately recast as one of intimacy characterized by reciprocity—where Hindu rajas were not considered rulers "as much as patrons who could serve their needs, receiving their cooperation in return."[13] The seasonal movement of Nakaro's ancestors had allowed them to graze in the waste areas and forestland that surrounded the villages and stretched up to the mountain passes.[14] They were even paid by peasants to settle in their fields nightly and provide manure.[15] To sustain this kind of movement, the Gaddi people had to be astute, market savvy, and distinctly visible. Women played a significant role in building relationships with local villagers, paying respect to the raja, and renewing deeds.[16] Families had multiple houses along grazing routes, and shepherds often had wives or mistresses in each house. Divorce was common, and women enjoyed relative sexual freedom, or at least the ability to have multiple partners over their lifetimes.[17] Though marriage was patrilocal, and wealth was concentrated in the hands of the head of the flock (*mahlundi*), the household structure was loose, involving neither nuclear nor extended joint families. Men and women both engaged in work in the fields and on the shepherding route, both negotiating business arrangements and taking wool and meat to market.

On the annexation of Punjab in 1849, G. C. Barnes, the first colonial district commissioner, began by privatizing communal lands and drawing distinct village and household units that could be managed for revenue extraction.[18] Gaddis found their access to forests closed, their rights redefined, their taxes increased, and the rhythms of their movements controlled by colonial administrators in a way that they had not been by their kingly patrons.[19] Nakaro's son, a former shepherd, explained:

> When there was a king, we used to pay him. Then, a new ruler came with the colonial administration. The forest department was made, we were totally dependent on the forest and now we had to pay for it. If we had a hundred sheep, the forest officer would come to the house twice per year and count our animals and require us to pay tax and get a permit. If someone complained, then they would come and fine them, the permits were not fixed. In the old times [under the raja], if we had a permit, they didn't even count, there was a system of trust.

Under colonial administration, demand for timber changed the use of forest resources, meaning Gaddis were seen as a burden on the state as opposed to a rich revenue source. Gaddi herders began to migrate down to the foothills of Kangra, originally as bonded laborers (*pahgiri*). As mentioned in chapter 1, fears that the new land market would be dominated by wealthy outsiders were addressed with the introduction of the Punjab Alienation of Land Act of 1900, which prohibited members of castes classified as nonagricultural from buying land from agricultural castes. This promoted agriculture as a more respectable profession than shepherding, deepening divisions between caste groups that had previously been less pronounced.[20] Unlike lower castes who were forced into waged employment, Gaddi Brahmins and Rajputs, such as Nakaro's family, were classified as agricultural, and hence they were able to purchase additional land without competition by selling their flocks.[21] As such, they were able to establish themselves as small landowners and began to engage in cash cropping. With a view to reducing their flocks, the state doubled taxation on Gaddi herders between 1915 and 1917.[22] John Middleton, the commissioner at the time, suggested even more "repressive" measures in the form of outright restrictions on the number of sheep any shepherd could have.[23]

The process of land enclosure was paralleled by a process of domestic enclosure that shifted the domestic division of labor. In the early Settlement reports, colonial administrators were struck by the freedom of sexuality and mobility that women enjoyed. Barnes observed in 1855, "Generally, women in the lower hills take no part in agriculture, confine themselves to the domestic occupation of breadmaking, fetching water and all the field work devolves to males. About Kangra, the population consists of a lower caste, structurally agricultural and here the women work as hard, if not harder than their husbands. The men drive the plough and the harrow, sow the seed, and thresh out the corn, and the women carry out and distribute the manure, crush the clods, weed the fields and carry home the harvest."[24]

Kriti Kapila's readings of archival evidence "against the grain" suggest that both colonial administrators and publics were alarmed by the sexual and marital practices that underpinned this loose domestic division of labor and household structure.[25] As Kapila details, in April 1879 the secretary of state for India noticed a statement in the selections from the vernacular newspapers published in Upper India that a "slave trade prevails in Kangra district of the Punjab and that not only are women publicly bought and sold but there is an office of the deeds of sale." Clarification from the governor of Punjab came in the form of a report from the assistant district commissioner, who clarified that this was not a slave trade but a system whereby a conjugal relation could be severed, initiating divorce and remarriage through a payment from one man to another, critically *with* the consent of the woman in question. He notes that "conjugal affection is not deep" in the region and that "morals are extremely loose here, and the standard of civilisation so low that it is to be feared that the infidelity of wives is the rule rather than the exception."[26] Between 1855 and independence in 1947, district commissioners used legal strictures to consolidate the patriarchal line of inheritance, stigmatize divorce, and codify marriage (especially disincentivizing widow remarriage, or *karewa*). Kapila writes, "Over time, the Gaddi household became a reduced and a pared down version of itself, as more and more people became educated into a particular ideal of filial loyalties. The practical consolidation of this household ideal took hold and filial emotion was constrained by these laws and reinterpreted in the idiom of 'blood.' If in earlier times, services to a person during her or his lifetime may have eventuated in a share of their property, such transfers were getting more and more informed by the language of contractual reimbursements in the new legal definition of the family."[27]

THESE FORMS OF LAND and domestic enclosure did not result in an immediate transition but were a catalyst for a century-long shift in land-use arrangements, income generation strategies, domestic economy, and moral values for the Gaddis.[28] By the time of independence in 1947, the threat to the agropastoral economy intensified with further opportunities in slate mining, the lure of state-provided education, and the dramatic increase in population and habitation in the Kangra valley, restricting the land and labor available for either pastoralism or agriculture. In this immediate postindependence period, upper-caste Gaddis in Kangra were not recognized as Scheduled Tribes for their pastoral livelihood and were considered another agricultural caste. Their relationship to the new postcolonial state—including their retention of land and grazing rights, as well as the regulation of marriage, inheritance, and divorce—was mediated by provisioning under Kangra customary law. Such customary law was based on manuals compiled by district, determined by a principle of territoriality, which in turn was based on colonial topography and Settlement reports.[29] As a result, Gaddis in Kangra were determined to have more customary likeness to their territorial neighbors than to their kin in Chamba.

As detailed in the previous chapter, the project of integration for marginalized tribes began in the early 1970s under the Himachal Pradesh Tenancy and Land Reform Act 1972. This further promoted the uptake of agriculture in Kangra and invited Gaddis down the valley to take up new opportunities in agriculture. Following the First Indo-Pakistani War in 1971, the Gaddis were enfolded into military recruitment drives that were promoted across Himachal Pradesh. Many now-retired Gaddi ex-servicemen across castes had enlisted in this period—particularly in the Gorkhana and Rajputana Rifles regiments—seeking employment and social benefits, as well as respectability. The late 1970s and 1980s also saw the introduction of major road, hydroelectric, and dam infrastructural projects to the region, which created opportunities for waged employment. Infrastructural projects also promoted the growth of the tourism industry in the region, motivated both by the natural beauty of the region and by Hindi and Buddhist pilgrimage given the proximity to the Dalai Lama in McLeod Ganj and to major Hindu sacred sites.

As Gaddis took up sedentary agriculture or waged labor in these emergent sectors of the Kangra economy, the female contribution to household income became less visible and devalued, and women had less of a say in marital and divorce practices. They were no longer instrumental in productive activities such as tending to the flock or spinning wool. Instead, new norms of femininity that aligned with Kangri upper-caste Rajputs and Brahmins became critical to shedding their historical position as bonded laborers in the plains. As Gaddi families settled in Kangra and gave up their pastoral livelihoods, they came face-to-face with new kinds of patriarchal norms exhibited by their Pahari neighbors.[30] Particularly for Gaddi upper-caste men, it became necessary to exhibit greater authority over their wives and daughters to secure social prestige. Normatively, this meant the rise of female seclusion in the home, the practice of *ghoonghat* (sexual avoidance and veiling in front of one's husband's male relatives), and the withdrawal of women from waged employment. This did not mean women ceased to work altogether but that they engaged in subsistence agriculture and animal husbandry (keeping cows or goats), which came to be considered housework. As such, women came to be considered a sexual risk and an economic burden on the households of their fathers and, subsequently, their husbands.

NAKARO WAS BORN INTO these new gendered conditions. She doesn't know exactly when but thinks it must have been just after independence. She didn't go to school and was thirteen when she married. It was not until some years later, past the brink of puberty, that she moved to the low fields of her husband's village. Nakaro's mother-in-law was a notoriously formidable woman—enterprising, quick-witted, cunning. Even today, stories are told of her political skill in negotiating land use with local village leaders, making astute deals as she sold her husband's wool or meat. She herself had spent her life on the shepherding route—her own father was a very wealthy herdsman. After eleven pregnancies she maintained her health and vigor. Indeed, as Nakaro conceived her first daughter, her mother-in-law conceived her last child. Her elder four children took on the family's livelihood as shepherds and, as such, remained illiterate and uneducated. The eldest daughter married into another eminent shepherding family and to this day maintains the family's land in Chamba. They still have a house there, perched on the hill overlooking the village, where they maintain a grove of walnut trees and fields of red kidney beans. The eldest son inherited his mother's business acumen, initially brokering deals with Tibetan merchants in the wool markets of Dharamsala and Palampur before moving into the business of land purchase and sale. Nakaro's husband had his mother's charisma and gravitas and, as his elder brother showed no interest in the hard work of shepherding, took on the responsibility for the flock by securing not only his father's grazing permits but also those of his uncles.

Nakaro's family purchased land in Kangra when her eldest sons were born. Before this, their family would stay as bonded laborers in Kangra, escaping the bitter Chamba winter. As they crossed through Dharamsala, they worked the fields of a Brahmin family. When they moved further south to the plains, they harvested the fields of a Hindu Gujjar family in the Shivalik hills. They sold their whole flock to purchase agricultural land of their own in a village south of Dharamsala, the first of many times during Nakaro's husband's life that they would be forced to sell their livestock. On this land they built a mud house in which, over the course of his life, their family would spend more and more time until the nomadic lifestyle of the family would fade into memory. Nakaro's mother-in-law had different aspirations for her younger children and particularly great hopes for her younger daughters. They were educated and matched with men with brighter futures that took advantage of the influx of money into the region. They would not be shepherding wives but housewives to men who could provide for them.

Nakaro's children have told me of the violence that Nakaro suffered when she moved into her marital home. Villagers remember seeing her flee up to the tops of trees, blood running down her face. Initially this abuse was part of the normal pattern of household authority—a new bride was obligated to serve her husband's family. Then Nakaro failed to produce a son. She had first one, then two, then three daughters, and the violence worsened. Nakaro's children were seen as unclean, uneducated, and uncivilized by their kin and neighbors because they still went with their father on the shepherding routes. Local doctors encouraged her to leave her husband and her marital family. Finally, for some time in the 1980s, she took her youngest son and went back to live in her *maike* (natal home). They took her in with kindness, but the pressure to return grew, and she went back.

* * *

THROUGHOUT THE COURSE OF his life, Nakaro's husband was caught between his wife and his sisters. Indeed, Nakaro's children would often remark on how different their parents were. Where Nakaro was independent and withdrawn, Arjun was almost compulsively social—along the shepherding route, he was known for his quick, sarcastic tongue and warm heart. Where Nakaro's sense of self was drawn from her work, Arjun was aesthetic and proud, emanating the elegant masculinity of Gaddi men. Arjun enchanted me just as he had enchanted slate miners and shepherds alike on the grazing pastures. In May and in November, when he was crossing through the village with his herd, he would come to visit me. On these mornings I was awoken at first light by a knock on my door. Arjun would climb our stairs slowly in his rubber shoes, the slow, steady step of a hill man. Even at this hour, after walking hours down from the *dera* (campsite) carrying heavy loads of goat milk or meat, he would be dressed immaculately: a crisp beige or gray kurta and pyjama, the distinctive coatee of the Gaddis—coarse goat hair handwoven so thickly, so tightly, that it is waterproof—fastened with gleaming buttons and cut high in the Nehru style around his neck. An embroidered Gaddi *topi* (hat) was perched and tilted on the crown of his head. On these mornings when he came down from the mountains, he often had his gun slung over his shoulder. He had a face weathered by years of crossing the high passes. His features were typically Gaddi—small slit-like eyes, an arresting nose that was slightly off-kilter, having been broken years ago. He would chide me for being lazy, for sleeping in. I would rush to get him a comfortable seat and serve him hot tea—always in a steel cup, for he felt uncomfortable with fancy bone china. He would slurp his tea, take a biscuit. I would have a few small packets of *beedi* waiting for him. He would pull one out and savor the first burn at the back of his throat.

Nakaro and Arjun mapped their personal history to that of the mountains. The slow looping of the grazing route mirrors the ups and downs of their life. Their histories were marked by long stretches of separation, loneliness, moments of extreme sociality, and a steadily increasing sense of hardship as the mountains filled up, leaving less space for their flocks. Significant points in their lives are plotted by the places, ridges, temples, streams, and mountains. The Chamba Nag (snake) temple where they had sought the blessing of a son after the birth of their three eldest daughters and two miscarriages, before eventually being rewarded with two healthy boys. The *dhar* (shepherding hut) high in the forestland of the Kangra hills, where Nakaro came to take refuge from the violence with her children and where they spend every monsoon to this day. The noxious lantana, an invasive weed that began to creep up the hillsides, devouring the pristine grasslands, herbs, and flowers that sustained their herd. The great scar at the foot of the hills where the slate mines are, providing Arjun with petty work while he rebuilt his herd after selling them to buy his own land in Kangra. The twist in the road where, while Arjun slept, his three hundred sheep and goats were stolen, rustled onto the back of a truck by thieves from the plains. The high valley where, when the snow came late, he was left stranded in the high pastures, and when the rains came early, his herd was washed down the river.

As the hardships of shepherding grew more challenging for Arjun, so too did the hardships of the household for Nakaro. Her skills became increasingly redundant. There is no longer any need to go with her husband and the herd, to help with the birthing of the kids or with the crossing of difficult places, for Arjun keeps only fifty sheep and goats now. Even if he kept more, it would be cheaper to hire a Punjabi migrant worker. There is no longer any need to spin coarse wool into yarn to be sold at the market, nor to weave thick *pattu* (blankets) from the yarn—Tibetans buy the wool of the cheaper Rajasthani goats, and hand looms are considered cumbersome. There is no need to grow seasonal vegetables and subsistence crops of wheat, corn, and lentils when they can be bought more cheaply from the market, subsidized by the government below-poverty-line card they are entitled to because of their Scheduled Tribe status. As her husband's flock decreases in size year by year, his contribution to the household wanes, as does her own. Instead, the bulk of the household income comes from their children. Their daughter is married to a military man. Their eldest son now has a steady government job and is on his way to completing his own MA in computer studies. Even their youngest son, after twelve years of shepherding with his father, gave up the profession, painfully, to begin his own paragliding business after their herd was stolen for a second time by thieves in the Punjab plains. In their new house, recently built from concrete on new land purchased for their eldest son's nuclear family, Nakaro and Arjun look anachronistic. Often unable to sleep in the raised beds given to them, they curl up by the fire in the kitchen or can be found creeping back to their old, deserted mud house to sit on the low balcony that overlooks the fields. Nakaro's commitment to keeping this house clean and the farm well-kept—applying fresh *lipai* (dung paint) every season, dusting, sowing, harvesting—goes largely unnoticed.

Nakaro herself explained how the enclosure of common land had impacted her life one day while we were sitting by the river watching her cow graze. Looking out at the opposite riverbank, she spoke of a time when all women used to come and graze their animals in the afternoon by the river. It was a time to share news, feelings, and friendships. As fewer women keep animals now, the margins of common land decrease, and women are pushed into their homes, where mobility is restricted. Indeed, Nakaro's life has been marked by a shift in the division of labor in her household, where women have withdrawn from productive labor and taken up positions as housewives. Nakaro has lived this devaluation of female productive labor and witnessed the rise of a new world into which she does not quite fit. The change has driven Arjun to drink. Beginning with a habit to fight the cold and hardship of the nomadic life, he, like many elder men of the village, has come to drink daily. The more Arjun drinks, the more her children neglect her, the more Nakaro sees herself as *kamzor*.

Loss of *Dharam*, Loss of Substance

The life history of Nakaro and Arjun illustrates the deep existential uncertainty that has come with the loss of pastoralism and the destruction of the landscape. This uncertainty permeated the terrain, household, and body. As chapter 1 explored, this is felt as a rise in jealousy, witchcraft, and illness. This is attributed by many to a change in *dharam* that had come with a loss of pastoral livelihoods. *Dharam* is a relational term that indicated both the mixing and separation of substances and sentiments between people and the land that came through a particular form of *kaam*, or labor. As Alf Hiltebeitel put it, the Sanskrit word *dharma* means that which "holds" or "upholds." It can also be translated as "foundation," in that a foundation is something that holds. He suggests that here it is opposed to other terms such as *nirvana* and *moksa*, both of which describe the goal of liberation—where liberation "usually has to do not with 'holding' but with 'letting go.'"[31]

The Gaddi woman's role in holding moral life was further explained by Deepak, an elderly Gaddi Brahmin, one hot May afternoon in the courtyard of his home. "Fifty years back, we were the people in the mountains," he told me. "We were totally self-sufficient. The women were the keepers of this *dharam*." Deepak lounged lazily on the daybed, propping his head up on a spindly arm. His mustache and nose hairs were neatly trimmed, and his graying hair was combed flat on his spotted scalp with mustard oil. He waited for his daughter-in-law to leave her work chopping leaves for her goats. She greeted us, pulling her scarf low over her face. Once we were settled with steaming tea, he checked his gold watch, twisted the gemstone on his middle finger, and looked me straight in the eye. "*Dekho* [look]," he said, "I'll tell you." He launched into a monologue that would take us well beyond our agreed meeting time:

> I am speaking about one hundred years ago; now we have had freedom [from the British] for seventy years. I am seventy-two years old. I am talking about things that have happened in my lifetime. Our ancestors

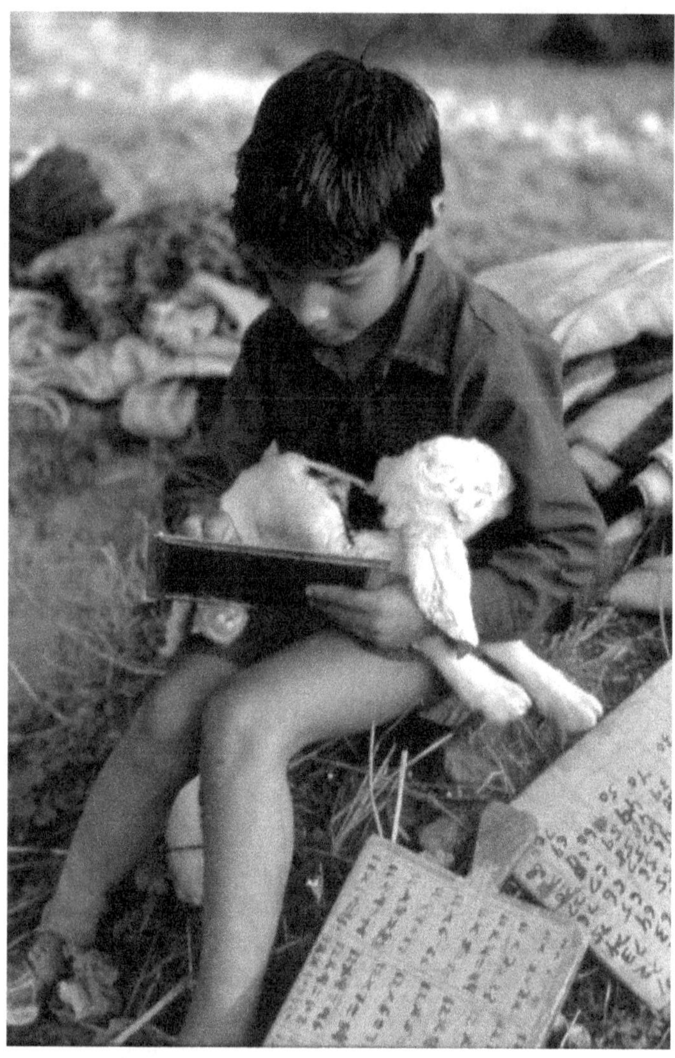

FIGURE 2.3. A young Gaddi boy studying on the shepherding trail. Photograph by Tejinder Singh Radhawa, 1980.

were uneducated. . . . Mountain people who ate simple food and made woolen things to cover themselves. . . . People had to work to fill their stomachs. There weren't any special government schemes to provide work. But now it is a new scientific age, and everyone has left that old lifestyle—the young generation is all studying. Now they are doing learned jobs and will earn seventy thousand to eighty thousand [rupees] per month, they will eat, and they buy everything. They will not make their own things. They are forgetting their culture. They depend on others.

In Deepak's complaints we find a narrative typical of an elder generation of Gaddi upper-caste men that frames ecological destruction—depletion of grassland, poisoning of soil—as simultaneous to the rupture of relationships between kin, between humans and animals. The strategic essentialism in the depiction of Gaddi *dharam* by Deepak reveals a particular kind of "Hindu worlding" that was present in many upper-caste Gaddi narrations. As Arkotong Longkumer puts it, such "Hindu worlding" is where natural images and metaphors are used to reinscribe and sacralize relations among people, animals, nature, deities, and the universe according to a broader Hindu national imaginary and rubric of Indic civilization.[32] During my fieldwork among the Gaddis this worlding had not involved explicit activist campaigns or violence. However, Deepak's narrations speak to a broader upper-caste discourse that asserts patriarchal gendered norms and casted hierarchies *within* the broader project of Hinduizing tribal religion and relations to land. This discourse itself is not rigidly ideological, nor does it follow a straightforward script of nationalism or Sanskritization; instead, it is porous and malleable, allowing seemingly conflictual projects of tribal self-determination or rural self-making to be enfolded within.[33] The ways in which such ideology permeates everyday worlds are diverse and include being a vegetarian, watching Hindu epics on television, visiting temples, sharing religious WhatsApp content, and reworking household and communal ritual practices such as the Gaddi *nuala* (Shaivite animal sacrifice ritual). However, the domain into which anxieties were often displaced was that of respectability (*izzat*), and particularly the sexual behavior of young women.[34] Deepak continued:

In the new generation, the [mental] changes that have happened to girls have been caused by the control of society. We and our society try to control them and put pressure, because they aren't able to live like we did in the old times. We want them to live with *izzat*. We lived like that because we feared our parents and respected them. In those times, people

> were very uneducated and respected each other. When they are all educated, they become more cunning. Girls particularly, they want their own "things." Now girls are all out of our hands. But if we're not able to give them those things, then they'll run away. They think that if they live like us, then they will become *duffer* [useless]. If they live in their own way, then we'll become *duffer*.

Where elderly men were especially concerned with younger generations' lack of respectability and eschewal of patriarchal authority, elderly women were more concerned with the obsolescence of their *kaam*. "There is no time to rest," Nakaro told me one day when we were walking through the wheat fields in the village. "My life has been very hard; we women are always working." Elderly women like Nakaro explained that they had become *kamzor* because they had done and were still doing too much *kaam*, and as a result, *kamzori* had accumulated in their bodies over time. *Kaam* is usually used to refer to petty waged or informal labor, in opposition to *naukri*, or formal employment. Yet, in its more expansive emic sense, *kaam* refers to any kind of labor—productive, caring, or ritual—that generates or sustains life. Such labor is the application of *shakti*, or life force, to the world. As such, the products of one's *kaam*—whether they be the fruits reaped from agricultural or pastoral labor, the relationships within a household, or the products of housework—are imbued with this vital force.[35] The word *kaam*, for elderly women, referred to productive labor—marked by endless hard physical work that they had to do in the fields, caring for animals, a condition that their daughters did not have to endure given the withdrawal of respectable housewives from the fields. It also referred to reproductive and caring labor—household work such as cleaning, cooking, sewing clothes, spinning wool without the support of modern appliances—and to the literal reproductive work of birth and childrearing.

Elderly women drew attention to the backbreaking *kaam* that they had performed throughout their lives, hardship that was not experienced or honored by upwardly mobile younger generations. This hardship was acute for elderly widows or women whose husbands had not secured profitable land, military, or formal employment but instead engaged in precarious waged work as laborers or slate miners. Parvana, a Gaddi widow, reflected that when her children were young, her husband died suddenly, and there was no way of getting resources for the family. "I had to go and work in people's houses, then after that go to the fields to work. While I was working, I had to watch over the children, so I had to take them with me. . . . The children's lives were bad, and my life was bad." But now, Parvana said, her children do not experience this kind of precarity. As a result of her hard work, they were able to go to school and now earn an income in good jobs instead of having to work for others or do farming. Parvana was proud of this achievement, but she also felt it was not acknowledged.

Gaddi women's anxieties about younger generations tended to focus on their daughters and daughters-in-law. They were concerned that their sons marry educated women to improve their status, while simultaneously fearing their daughters-in-law would not continue to perform *dharam*. They lamented that younger generations did not do the domestic, agricultural, and ritual *kaam* that they had done, aspiring instead to middle-class domestic practices, tertiary education, or the pursuit of business opportunities. Young women even took on different forms of ritual labor—neglecting the care of traditional household gods and instead engaging in mainstream Hindu practices such as *karwa chauth*, a day of fasting and prayer for their husbands, or praying to Hindu gods like Ganesh who were not worshiped by generations before. Reena, a Gaddi woman in her seventies, chuckled cynically at the thought of fasting for the "useless, drunken fool" that was her husband and giving up a day of work. The discontinuity of ritual labor had great significance, as it was traditionally a woman's role to transmit female substance to future generations through worship of household gods.[36] Elder women often failed to appreciate the financial and social strains on young women, whom they saw as caught up instead in exchanges on social media, watching soap operas, and always "running back to their natal home." They were often piqued that younger women didn't acknowledge the hardships that previous generations had gone through to accumulate wealth.

Anxieties relating to the loss of *dharam* and the hardship of unacknowledged *kaam* were often discussed through bodily change. For this elder generation, the landscape was the primary source of vitality, and their bodies were considered to consist of the substances drawn from that place.[37] Health was largely associated with having good blood (*khun*), which in turn comes from compatible foods grown on the land.[38] Many spoke of the times before, when Gaddi bodies had strength, fitness, and agility as a result of *kaam*—communion with the landscape and animals. People ate the fresh, nourishing meat of goats grazed on flowers and herbs, as well as homegrown seasonal vegetables, and they drank healing goat milk. They had been able to climb the mountains with ease and to resist the cold, wind, and rain.

With sedentarization, the rhythms of Gaddi bodies have changed, and the authoritative claim to the landscape has been diluted. Most waged work is not considered by elderly people to be a source of *shakti*. Elderly women lamented that their daughters were unable even to climb to the high hills above the village to cut grass for their animals, as their bellies had become swollen by daily consumption of rice. Habituation to foods that were supposed to generate heat in the body, like alcohol and onions, had spoiled blood and demeanor, leaving people with overt passions, lust, and aggression. These qualities were said to result in alcoholism and violence for men and sexual impropriety for women. The body was further spoiled by the consumption of vegetables from the market and ruined by "dependence" on the "poisoned" foods sprayed with pesticides that were imported from Punjab. Such foods were the cause of new kinds of ailments unseen before, including kidney stones and gallstones, forms of cancer and heart disease, disrupted digestive processes, and jaundice. Elderly people who could still feed their families from the fresh meat of their own herds and homegrown vegetables saw themselves as healthier than and morally superior to their neighbors.

This generalized state of bodily disruption caused by the loss of *dharam* was the backdrop against which more acute complaints of *kamzori* were made. *Kamzori* was a loss of vitality, a low ebbing frequency that permeated households that had transitioned away from agricultural or pastoral work, whose intergenerational relations were fraught with conflict. It depleted the bodies of elderly women who had experienced a lifetime of hardship and hard work—women who had alcoholic husbands, who were widowed early in their lives, or who had lost out on land. Men who experienced such fraught situations were more likely to directly blame their kin for inadequate care or respect. In women's stories of *kamzori*, blame was assigned obliquely, and etiologies slipped between environmental, domestic and intimate causes.

I encountered *kamzori* in the body of Jugaan, who had supported her husband with the herd all her life. She had come to complain of *kamzori* and searing headaches around the time she was trying to find her son a suitable bride. I encountered it in Rinky, who became afflicted with *kamzori* and jaundice (*piliya*) when her son and his wife migrated to Delhi to take up waged work, leaving her alone and unable to manage her household or to keep the fields. I also saw it in Sarita, who explained that she had become weak, bedbound, and "soft-minded" soon after her daughter-in-law had "abandoned" her and become consumed with her own small tailoring business. I heard it from Rani, who was *kamzor* because her husband had become an alcoholic, leaving her to bring in money by working at a local construction site. In short, *kamzori* was an intimate, painful experience of disruption that occurred simultaneously in the body, in domestic relationships, and in the wider landscape. But not all women complained of bodily disruption and *kamzori*; indeed, some were content with the shift in life and livelihood.

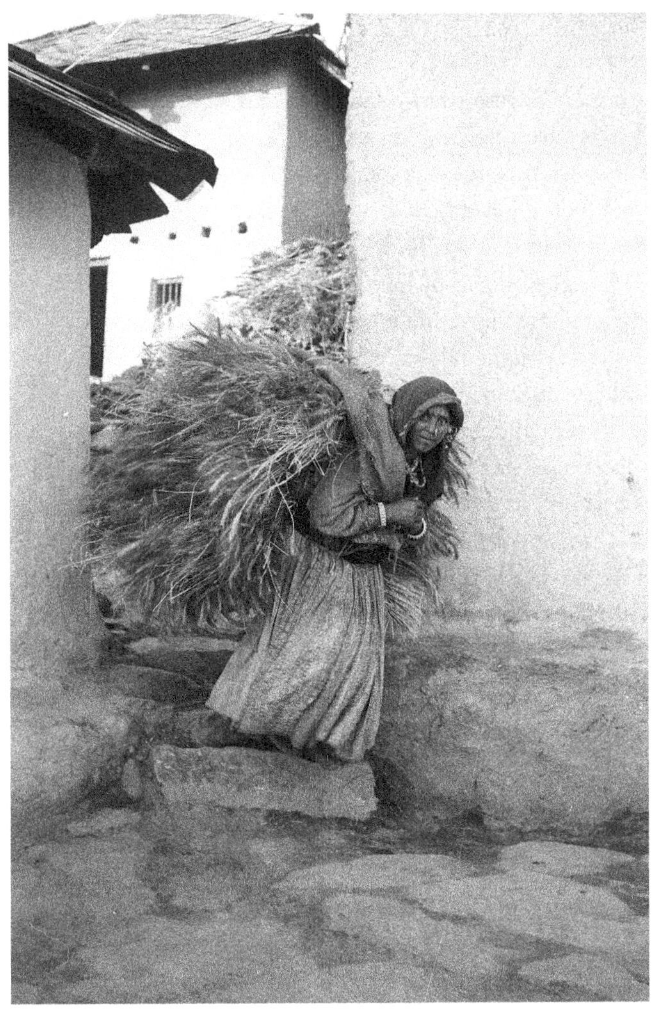

FIGURE 2.4. A Gaddi woman carries a heavy load of harvested wheat. She wears traditional Gaddi dress (*luanchiri*) with Rajasthani fabric and a *dora* (woolen rope) around her waist. Photograph by Peter Phillimore, 1977.

Two Women

I remember the ease with which Jagatambo held her thin frame, her legs folded beneath her, her arms casually draped over the top of her head. As a widow, she wore a simple white kurta, but somehow she seemed majestic as she sat, surrounded by her daughters-in-law on the ornate balcony of her son's palatial house. I met Jagatambo when I was in the midst of interviews with other widows of the village, weighed down by tales of financial insecurity. In contrast, Jagatambo welcomed me up freshly tiled stairs to a daybed where she was having tea with her two daughters-in-law. She sat peacefully as I asked her about the loss of her husband some ten years prior. "It was normal." She waved her hand dismissively. "My children were there to help me and give me money." She explained that she had stopped wearing red, her favorite color, and begun to dress simply, but she still ate mutton and chicken even though this wasn't customary for widows. "Mum is the head of the house still!" Her daughter-in-law Radha chuckled affectionately. Jagatambo could rest as she had doting daughters-in-law who still tended fields of wheat and corn, cooked with homegrown ingredients, and carried out daily prayers for the household gods. Jagatambo was able to replace her material contribution to the household with the bestowal of blessings. "My children are always there for me," she explained when I asked who supported or cared for her. "I have thousands of friends as well." She spoke particularly of her dear friend who lived in nearby Palampur and mentioned that they were able to visit one another or speak regularly over the phone.

Midway through our interview, Jagatambo's son Surjeet entered, wearing a well-ironed shirt and thick gold chain. He had a fresh streak of vermilion and ash on his forehead, having just been to the temple. Later, Shankar whispered that Surjeet had done very well for himself as a businessman, a property dealer. Jagatambo's husband had been a shepherd, and she had even supported him on the shepherding route throughout her married life. When he died, Surjeet had sold the family's whole herd of sheep and goats for six lakh rupees and bought land in a Kangra village. The family gave up their seminomadic life and settled permanently so the younger members could go to school. Surjeet quickly sold this land for much more than he had paid for it and began a thriving property business. Sweeping his hand across the horizon, he showed me that he kept a great deal of land for subsistence and cash cropping. The women of the house, though dressed now in expensive suits, helped to sow and harvest these crops and kept a cow for daily fresh milk—honoring the wishes of their mother-in-law.

Jagatambo herself was able to withdraw from such work. She described her body as aging, but such descriptions appeared benign. Her contribution to the household might be increasingly obsolete, but her authority and wishes were still honored by her son, who provided financially, and her daughters-in-law, who were both caring and submissive. Such removal from labor was difficult for elderly women who, unlike Jagatambo, didn't trust the younger generation to secure the vitality of the household or provide adequate care. It involved stepping away from the lifetime of work they had done to build, sustain, and reproduce a household. This work was exhausting, but it was also foundational to their sense of self.

UNLIKE JAGATAMBO'S, NAKARO'S CHILDREN and daughter-in-law did less to honor her lifetime of hard work. The pain of such neglect came to a crescendo for Nakaro after Raman's wedding. When the festivities had ended, Nakaro left Raman's bride, Meena, alone. The family all moved into the new concrete house, but Nakaro looked out of place among the modern appliances. When she was in the new house, she spent most of her time in the separate mud kitchen, staring into the fire while she stitched together old rice bags to form pillows or picked the stones from dried lentils. She kept returning to clean the family's mud house each day, unaccompanied by her sons or daughter-in-law. It became clear that Meena was not interested in helping Nakaro tend to the horses or cut the wheat, or in climbing the foothills up to the family shepherding hut. Meena complained of a sore back and locked herself in her plush room, spending hours on the phone to her sisters. Nakaro did not chide her but instead resigned herself, crestfallen. Meena herself was concerned with securing a position with a local tailor so that she could earn some money. As the daughter of a businessman, she had never done the hard farmwork or trekking that this family was used to. Her family no longer worshipped a household god, so she looked blank when Nakaro explained how she worshipped a clan god instead of going to the Hindu temple.

Nakaro's complaints of *kamzori* grew acute when the atmosphere of the household was particularly fraught. She described the condition as a chronic sense of bodily depletion that caused her to lose her strength. Sometimes, around moments of family conflict, her condition swelled into fever, insomnia, or muscle ache. In the height of summer, when the family had been living in the concrete house for some six months and Meena's disinterest in agricultural work had become apparent, Nakaro began to spend more and more time in the old mud house. One day she developed a high temperature. The night before, she hadn't slept at all. She complained that she couldn't sleep in the new concrete house. I lay beside her on the balcony of the mud house. Her son threw a thick blanket over us, despite the summer heat. When she closed her eyes, she would see trees, a concrete house, lights like in a wedding, a lot of needles, a flower garden, lots of people—lots and lots of people—women she didn't know. They came to her in flashes, and her thin body twitched. The fields were beautiful, she told me. But maybe they were so beautiful because she had been cursed by *opara*; maybe there was something inside of her, she muttered. She told me, "I am thin and *kamzor*, and since I have moved to this new [concrete] house, I have been ill. I haven't had any health problems in my life. But now I just have this *kamzori*." The next day, I tried to take her to the hospital. In its cavernous corridors, she looked even more disoriented. "My main problem can't be solved here in the hospital because I know what it is. It is *kamzori*." She waved her hand dismissively—the condition, she told me, rendered her body resistant to medication. Still, when we returned home, even though she was feverish, she went to the fields to work. She said it was only through such work that she might find her strength again.

A Waning Life

When women like Jagatambo received the wealth, care, and respect they thought they deserved in these new domestic and economic conditions, they did not tend to experience premature symptoms of *kamzori* and were able to age peacefully. Here, successful aging was associated with strong relations of care within the household and a retention of domestic authority, as well as with the ability of an elderly person to benefit from the present circumstances of market integration, such as land possession, prestige marriage, or wealth accumulation. Indeed, the ability of younger generations to honor the livelihoods and wishes of their elders was, to some extent, dependent on their wealth gained outside the pastoral economy. Intergenerational relations were facilitated by favorable economic circumstances and the willingness on the part of younger generations to rework traditional ideas of Gaddi respectability into patterns of eldercare.

For women like Nakaro, who felt that their relationship to work and place had been severed and who did not receive care and respect in their new homes, complaints of *kamzori* and its associated ailments proliferated. These forms of bodily weakness were not blamed directly on family members or the loss of domestic authority, and sufferers did not attribute distress directly to vast forces like urbanization. Instead, the condition expressed subtler tensions in domestic relations of care and a more diffuse anxiety about ecological destruction, the devaluation of women's labor, conditions of housing, ritual piety, their children's employment prospects, or the challenges of the marriage market. For example, even though the acute symptoms associated with Nakaro's *kamzori* flared up during family conflict and in relation to Meena's behavior, she attributed the condition to the concrete house and the general hardship she had experienced over the course of her lifetime. It was not Meena's specific refusal to work in the fields or to come to the shepherding hut that necessarily offended Nakaro, but a more general melancholic sense that such work was not valued by a younger generation and hence that Meena did not show appreciation for the contribution Nakaro had made to the household by honoring Nakaro's wishes.

Here, care for the elderly is not only physical care or even respect but a wider intergenerational ethics of acknowledgment, attentiveness, and appreciation of mundane sacrifice that has been made over a lifetime. As Maya Mayblin observes among Santa Lucian women in northeastern Brazil who have experienced great hardship, this sacrifice is not easily located in classic anthropological terms because, rather than constituting an "event," it is more of a lived aesthetic—a generative mode of being-in-the-world.[39] We might read this approach into other examples of gendered bodily weakness in the anthropological record. Claire Snell-Rood's interlocutors, for example, women living in a Delhi slum, cited weakness as a bodily condition that resulted from emotional and physical endurance. One interlocutor, Geeta, explained, "Women have to endure the sadness of everything. . . . They are weak [*kamzor*] so that if they have eaten, if they take medicine, they won't even feel its impact."[40] The condition was produced by both their excessive caregiving responsibilities and the lack of reciprocal care that they received from others. Similarly, Sabina Rashid points out that married women living in Bangladeshi informal settlements also speak of the weakness (*durbolota*) that family care embeds in their bodies. She links weakness to the condition of *dhatu rog*, or white discharge, that many of these women also report. Lack of care—including good food, hygiene, and comfort—results in the boundaries of the body becoming increasingly permeable, causing vitality, in this case literally in the form of white discharge, to leak out.[41]

We also see interesting parallels between *kamzori* and conditions of distress experienced by elderly women beyond South Asia, robbed of their rest in old age by shifts in the domestic cycle. Kristin Yarris shows us how Nicaraguan grandmothers use the condition of rumination—*pensando mucho*—to express the moral ambivalence of economic remittances as they struggle to care for their grandchildren while their daughters migrate.[42] Clara Han shows how elderly women in Chile are left to care for their children as they experience poverty and substance abuse, causing elderly women to become afflicted by nervous conditions and searing headaches as their sacrifice to their nation goes uncompensated.[43] Julie Livingston shows how the rise of chronic illness in Botswana renders elderhood longer but more fraught, where physical weakness marks social disempowerment rather than aggregated authority as it once did.[44] In these examples, we see the culturalist analysis of the aging body in a new light—at once revealing the intimate concerns of domestic relations and holding broader temporalities and spatialities of structural change.

Kamzor bodies hold time—the *longue durée* of history, the cyclical time of work, the fraying time of aging, the fractured time of generation. This historical approach to *kamzori* can be found elsewhere. Lawrence Cohen writes of the senility, *hath pair* (nonfunctional hands and feet), and impotence that mar the latter years of his lower-caste Camar interlocutors in Banaras. For these people, *kamzori* is a response to a lifetime of caste and class oppression framed by a longer history of coloniality.[45] People are weak because they are old but also because they are poor and stigmatized and because they have "bad families." As such, the condition offers sufferers a way of obliquely speaking about oppressive social hierarchies, while preserving their moral integrity. Saiba Varma also finds *kamzori* in the halls of a psychiatric institution in Kashmir, where the condition rendered visible the psychic impact of ongoing occupation that could not be treated as trauma or evidenced by technological imaging and that persisted in the presence of biomedical care.[46]

In Gaddi women's *kamzori*, the sacrifice of time is felt in the body and marked to others as a depletion of bodily substance, substance that should be provided through such care or acquired through this increasingly obsolete *dharam* and *kaam*. As such, women did not seek rest, medication, or biomedical care in *kamzori* but instead tended to do *more* work in the fields or the household in an attempt to recuperate lost vitality. Women like Nakaro returned endlessly to sow fields that their families were no longer dependent on for flour, and to tend cows that their families no longer needed for milk. As Radhika Govindrajan notes of Pahari women in Uttarakhand, the labor with animals and the land is an enactment of true love, *prem*—devotion that allowed them to keep working, even if such labor was devalued by both men and the wider capitalist economy.[47] *Kamzori* allows sufferers to insist on the relationality of their own bodies and render visible the ways in which such relations, with kin, governments, landscapes, and medical systems, are nonreciprocal. As a frequency that links body, household, and landscape, *kamzori* speaks to the waning of wider forms of vitality as a result of ecological degradation, the cleavage of generations, atrophy of marital relations, shifts in sexual moralities, affinal abuse, religious and ritual change, changing diets and consumption patterns, and the rise of jealousy. *Kamzor* bodies have lived this history and now hold this history in wasting muscles and permeable minds.

Coda

For Nakaro, abundance was only truly left in one place—the *dhar* (shepherding hut) where she spent her monsoon summers, high up in the hills. It was only here, she said, that her feelings of *kamzori* would leave her, that she would be able to become strong again. "After we plant the corn," she told me, "we will go back there. It is such a beautiful place; it is our place, so peaceful [*shanth*]," she repeated. Sure enough, she left for the *dhar* as soon as the corn was in the ground. She was slower than usual—hard calluses had formed on the soles of her feet, rubbing against the sides of her plastic shoes. She carried one hand-stitched bag of supplies and a tattered blue rucksack that made a hump on her curved back.

We went to visit them in late October, only a few months before my departure from Kangra. We left at around three in the afternoon and began to climb as the heat of the sun turned into the autumnal evening. We arrived at the *dhar* late in the evening, as the sun was setting over the crest of the ridge. The *dhar* was set high in the mountains, on the last ridge before the tree line that broke up into the high passes. Looking down from the stone ledge that surrounded it, you could trace out the whole map of the village. The fields receded as the sun set and the lights of the hotels blinked on, showing the clusters of villages up into the high hills, like swarming fireflies that merged into the bright epicenter of Dharamsala town.

They had done up the *dhar* beautifully. When I entered it through the low door, I was struck by how different it looked from the last time I was there. Before, the floor and walls were cracked and entirely ripped up in places by visiting langur monkeys who mine the mud for salt. Dust had hung in the air, and rubbish left by unwelcome foreign campers had lain unburned in the fireplace. This time, it was neatly organized and replastered. The careful work of Nakaro and Arjun was evident in the detail, such that the room held a faded dignity. The *chulha* (stove) was painted smooth with a fresh layer of *lipai* (dung paint), with the bay below it neatly swept. There was a small posy of wildflowers in the nook to the right-hand side of the *chulha*, in the place where Nakaro sat, next to the salt, dried chilies, and ears of smoked corn. On the floor next to the *chulha*, two mats were laid out, made from stitched plastic rice bags. The right-hand one was for Nakaro, who would sit with her legs folded up near her ears while she cut and stirred and rolled. The left-hand one was for Arjun, where he chatted with visiting shepherd friends and smoked *beedis* between pegs of evening whiskey. His big knife lay alongside him, its wooden handle smooth from use; he sharpened the long, curved blade nightly before using it to cut firewood or meat. Along the back were shelves cut into nooks in the thick mud wall. One held necessities: a small tube of Carmex, a tub of moisturizing cream, three leaves of tablets, a mirror, trimming scissors and a packet of henna hair dye, a screwdriver, and a pocketknife. Hung next to this was a thin log, suspended with ropes from the wooden eaves, that served to hang the thick handwoven Gaddi blankets. On the far right-hand wall were three old oil drums, washed clean and refilled—one with last year's harvest of kidney beans, one with rice, and one with the ground whole wheat flour from the winter crop. Beside this lay a broken spinning wheel, cobwebbed in the corner.

Nakaro sat on one side of the *chulha* on a dirty old sheepskin, beginning to make tea for us. Somehow she looked more alive than I had ever seen her, crouched with her legs under her. Arjun sat on the other side in his long johns, a woolen beanie, and his coatee. His legs stretched out in front of us. Nakaro cooked dinner, slicing marrow she had harvested from in between the cornstalks that morning. She was completely absorbed in her work, so much so that she couldn't hear when we called to her softly. She absently recited mantras under her breath, "jai mata, jai shiva, jai ram." After we had eaten the spicy marrow around the fire, Nakaro lay down beside me. Her hollow cheeks were slightly fuller. As she lay there, she smiled her gummy smile and let her hand fall away from the stubs of her teeth. "How do you like our place?" she asked tenderly. I said many times that it was so beautiful. She smiled more widely, contentedly, and reached to hand me a corncob she had charred in the embers. She spoke of her wishes to spend more time with her daughters, of how much work they had to do for their husbands. She spoke of how she would bring her children to this *dhar* in their childhood, of how her daughters could climb up here in one hour, loaded with big sacks of supplies, though now they can't even make it to the slate mines only thirty minutes from the village. She spoke of the passing of time, of her hard life, wearily but with acceptance. That night we slept soundly, swaddled side by side in thick blankets. The next day she sent us home with a bag of corn, a bottle of goat milk, and a pot of vegetables for her son, which we would find again days later, untouched, in the fridge of the new concrete house.

3

Ghar ki Tension

WHY IS CARE SO OFTEN THE SOURCE OF DISTRESS?

Panchlo Devi

Panchlo lived across the road from Shankar, my research companion. When we passed by on our way to the vegetable seller, I would often spot her sitting out in her courtyard shelling peanuts, staring out from behind the bracken. She never spoke to us, only nodded respectfully as we tramped up the hill past her house on our daily rounds of visiting. She kept her hair tied back in a severe bun at the base of her neck. Her teeth protruded slightly. Her skin was smooth. Most strikingly, she had deep blue-green eyes. They were like no others that I had seen, not the light brown or even the turquoise-flecked green of some Gaddi women.

Panchlo was in her early forties. She was married to the eldest son of a Rajput family who had come over the passes from Chamba to Kangra a generation ago, seeking their fortune in the slate mines. While her father-in-law had sold

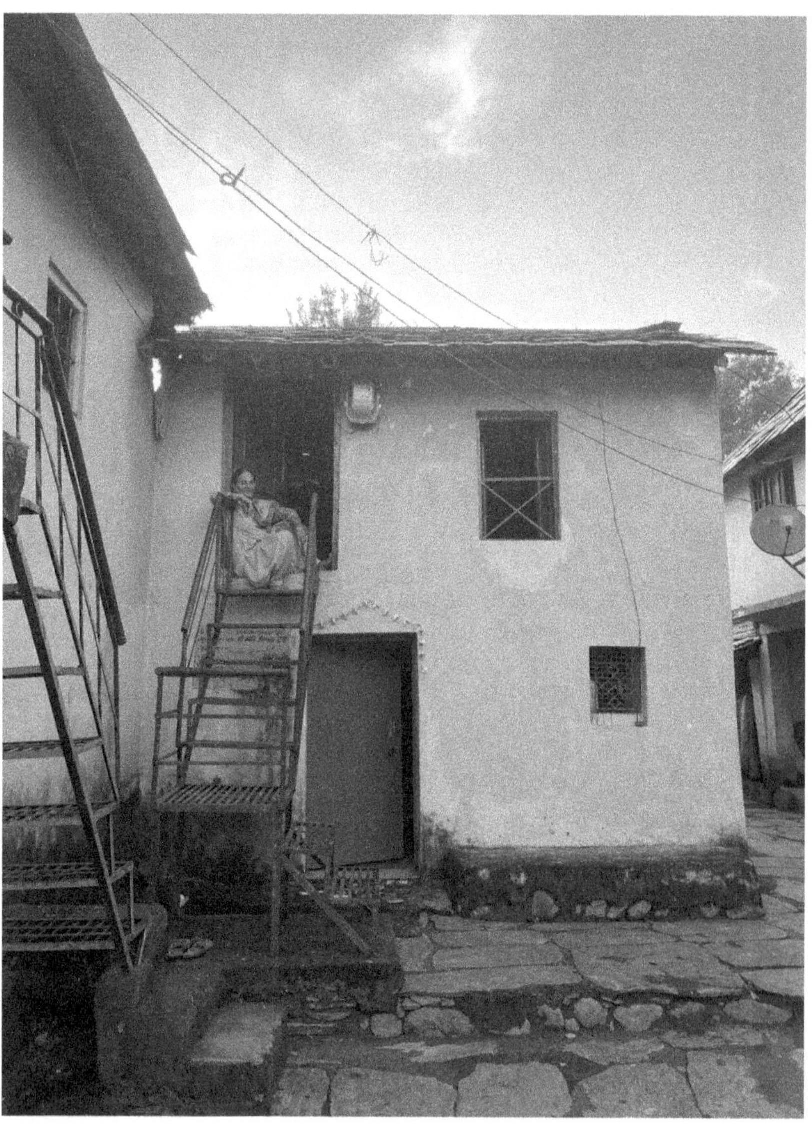

FIGURE 3.1. A Gaddi woman sits at the entrance to her kitchen. Photograph by Nikita Kaur Simpson, 2024.

their flock to chip slate until his death some five years ago, he had entertained great prospects for Panchlo's husband, the eldest of his three sons. Soon after Panchlo's wedding in 1996, her husband went to Delhi to work in a "private company," leaving her to care for his parents. She soon had two sons, conceived during his annual Diwali visits back to the village.

With her husband's monthly remittance payment, Panchlo was able to send her sons to the Lady of Mercy Catholic school in the nearby Tibetan settlement. As her sons grew into teenagers, the family moved out of the mud house that her in-laws had built when they settled in Kangra, for she was sick of the drudgery of sweeping the dry dirt from the floors, and the monthly labor of painting the floors with dung and patching cracks in the walls. She and her husband built a beautiful concrete house with a slate-paved courtyard. Lining the courtyard were soil beds that she grew fond of quietly tending in the time between breakfast and the lunchtime meal. In the beds she grew neat rows of garlic with tied tops, great bushes of the lemony coriander, and towering stalks of corn. Lining the beds she planted fruit trees—amla, apricot, and a particularly successful galgal tree from which she made a delicious pickle that her husband especially enjoyed when he came home from Delhi.

After an especially good year, when her husband's company gave him a small bonus, they built another story on the concrete house. The two-room set had an asbestos roof, a brown plastic bathroom, and a veranda that looked out over the Thera Road. Now it is rented more and more frequently by backpackers or techies from the cities who cross the road each day to set up in the new coworking space and café established by enterprising Brahmin neighbors. The rent money allowed Panchlo to send her elder son to college in Dharamsala, where he was struggling through a master's degree in computers. She never thought that in order to keep paying his fees, she would be forced to ask her neighbor for a job washing dishes in his café.

I first spoke properly with Panchlo on a blistering May afternoon. She gingerly invited me inside her home and into a small room off to the left side of the house. She offered me a plastic chair and curled up on the corner of the bed. It was one year after her husband had given up his job in Delhi and returned to their village. Panchlo told me that his return followed a leg and hip injury that left him hobbling through his office, unable to attend to the needs of clients and on some days paralyzed with pain. This pain drove him to drink: neat glasses of home-brewed rice spirit behind a curtain at the tea stall by the school.

What began as a habit became an addiction. Their wealth waned, and Panchlo was forced to find new ways of making money. She negotiated with neighbors to take care of their fields of wheat and corn in return for half the crop, which she could sell. She also began a milk business with her cow, selling to foreign neighbors. When I met her on that May day, Panchlo explained that the root of her problem is that she has to both earn money and care for the crumbling household. She kept her eyes fixed on a pair of shoes lying in the corner and picked at a loose thread in her chemise. The air between us was thickened by her worries: a declining income, college fees, a failed crop. She looked up at me directly and paused.

It was a familiar refrain: "Mujhe bahut ghar ki tension hai" (I have so much household worry), she sighed. "When my husband was OK, then it was OK. When he did a job and we made the house, then we used to joke around. The problem is that my husband can't work, and the burden [of earning and making household decisions] has come to me. Now the *bojh* [pressure, burden] has come to me. I have *ghar ki tension*. There is always *tension* when I try to go to sleep, and I think of the wheat—if it is outside, will it get wet? Because all the decisions are mine."

Panchlo doesn't worry only about her own household but also about how others see it. She feels ashamed of her struggles in her house and of her family's lack of security. "I just have one house, and other people have done so well compared to us; they have three or four houses, and we just have one house. I know that you must share [your *tension*]. But I don't like to share with anybody, I don't like to tell what is happening in my house; then they will talk. Also, everyone has their own tension, *apne ghar apne tension* [to each their house, to each their worries]." Panchlo worried that if others knew too much about her house, they would become jealous. Then they might be tempted to curse her with *opara*. She told me that her neighbors had already cursed her goats and her sheep, making them sick and even causing death. She had recently felt "*ghabrahat*—my heart going tuk tuk." This is the feeling one gets when one has been cursed by black magic. She sighed. "The *tension* I have is about my children, what will they do, what will they study. I have *ghar ki tension*. Then the result [of all this tension] is that you get all sorts of other illnesses." The space was laden with this *tension*. It was at once a feeling that Panchlo expressed, an embodied state, and an atmospheric mood. Panchlo felt this *tension* in her body, especially in its overheating. "When I have so much *tension*," she said, "I feel like just eating something and dying." She laughed nervously. "But then I picture my children there, and I think, who will look after them?"

The window into Panchlo's *tension* closed as quickly as it had opened. As I made my way from house to house, woman to woman, across Thera, this kind of window opened and closed time and time again. Though some women laughed it off, many needed only the gentlest probe—an inquiry about their marriage, the state of their finances, or their children's prospects—to be flooded with anxiety or to go to pieces. Their retellings of sicknesses, stretched household budgets, or alcoholic husbands felt like vain struggles to be free of a sticky web of worries.

While *tension* was used across the Gaddi community, it was primarily Gaddi married women who prefaced it with the qualifying *ghar ki* (household) to indicate a deeper disruption to bodily humors, intimate relations, and household materiality. *Ghar ki tension* spoke simultaneously to distressed relationships (marital discord, conflict with or within their husband's family or with their children), economic distress (food insecurity, lost employment), and physical distress (adverse reproductive events, the impact of household work and poor self-care on the body). Indeed, *ghar ki tension*, like *kamzori* (weakness), was a gendered form of distress. Married men did experience *tension*—I encountered numerous examples of men articulating the strain of providing for a family, smoothing conjugal relationships, and honoring the wishes of their parents or the expectations of their wider caste communities. However, there are three important differences to note about men's *tension*. First, the patriarchal nature of kinship relations meant that men, ultimately, did not see themselves as responsible for making and maintaining care relations, or managing distress within the household. Men were able to displace blame for *kharab* (bad) household *mahaul* (atmosphere) onto women. When they felt domestic frustrations, it was permissible and even encouraged to direct violence toward their wives in order to displace such responsibility. If women ever showed such violence, they would be considered unrespectable or even mad—as we will see in chapter 5. Second, men were mobile: When they experienced distress within the household, they were able to spend time outside of the domestic domain for work or leisure. They had access to vehicles, and their movements were not scrutinized. Third, men who experienced distress had access to a socially acceptable and even desired mode of release—alcohol.

Ghar ki tension was a feminized condition that existed in the materiality of the home and its atmosphere, and in the viscerality of a woman's body. The somatic expression of *ghar ki tension* was specific—it constituted a particular frequency of gendered distress. Where *kamzori*, as we saw in the previous chapter, was associated with the cooling of the body with aging and a loss of bodily strength, *ghar ki tension* was its opposite—a condition of hyperactivity in the body and the mind. *Ghar ki tension* was signaled by overheating of the body, unidentifiable aches, *high BP* (hypertension), insomnia, and rumination. Its sensation could also be concentrated in the heart and chest—associated with panic (*ghabrahat*) or feelings of suffocation. Women would suffer menstrual problems and abdominal pain. *Ghar ki tension* was also associated with malign forces—witchcraft (*jadu*), black magic (*opara*), and the evil eye (*nazar*)—entering the home through a woman's body. This occurred when the boundaries of the house and the woman's body became vulnerable to the envious gaze of kin and neighbors, causing serious illness.

Most often, what was at stake in women's expressions of *ghar ki tension* was care. It braided together the textured dilemmas and demands of ordinary care, and the critical events—death, disease, and violence—that punctuated the everyday. Women attributed their symptoms to constant housework and care work for ungrateful children, violent husbands, and demanding in-laws. They lamented moments when their husbands, in fits of rage, threw food that they had prepared. They complained of children who offered no help tending to fields or washing up after dinner. They decried endless tasks that surrounded the medical care of their fathers-in-law, or the interminable demands for massages, cups of tea, and hot rotis from mothers-in-law. It was not that they sought to resist these demands or shirk these responsibilities. On the contrary, most women took the greatest pride in keeping their homes clean and tidy and their household relations smooth—for this work was part of their ritual and even spiritual role in securing the well-being of the household. This caring labor gains greater importance as the Gaddi community aspires toward the lower rungs of India's middle class and seeks to accrue respectability.

Whereas their mothers and grandmothers grew up along the shepherding trail, a younger generation of Gaddi married women have reaped the benefits of profitable land sales and waged work, ushering them onto the lower rungs of India's middle class. For Gaddi women, obtaining middle-class status involved withdrawing from waged work, being able to depend on the secure income of a loving husband, and occupying oneself with the material, spiritual, and relational well-being of the house and those within it. Where their mothers and grandmothers looked backward toward a Gaddi past—holding the burden of lost knowledge and livelihoods in their bodies as *kamzori*—their daughters looked forward, aspiring toward a middle-class respectability that would secure their place in the nation and allow them to shed their reputation for tribal primitivism. As Hindu nationalism comes to frame this project, women's caring labor takes on an even deeper form of vitality. However, not all families have been able to benefit equally from this wave of economic prosperity. Those in secure formal employment such as military and government jobs (*naukri*) have had much smoother trajectories of social mobility than those in informal employ in the tourism, hydropower, and slate mining sectors. Women like Panchlo, whose husbands cannot earn, are faced with a contradiction between the material circumstances of their household and the pressure to cultivate its respectability. As they strive frustratedly toward middle-class respectability, these women are left with great burdens of care that often go unacknowledged by husbands, kin, and affines. Their predicament issues an even deeper question: Why is care so often a source of distress?

IN THE PREVIOUS CHAPTER, I looked at the ways in which bodies hold historical time in a context where a past immemorial seems to give way to a modern present. I argued that Gaddi elderly women feel anachronistic in this present, as their relational ties to the land and its vitalities, but also to younger generations, are truncated. The experience of *kamzori* expresses this wider rupture in generational time. Another way of thinking about this generational rupture is as the inability of elder and younger women to acknowledge one another's present. Their expectations of kinship, femininity, and care simply no longer match up. In this chapter I look at this rift from the perspective of the new generation of married women who have not grown up on the shepherding trail. For them, the present is not bounded by or oriented toward the past, but it still remains fraught. Why should that be, for a generation of women who seem to have nothing to lose?

I find Clara Han's definition of care useful for bringing into view time, relationality, and distress. Drawing on Stanley Cavell, Han defines care as the act of being, or becoming, present to another.[1] Herein, care is framed not as a category, a structure, or even as an intentional practice. Instead, care is a temporal problem of presence that becomes the subject of a moral dilemma. For Gaddi women, the moral dilemma of care is: How to be present to another, even an intimate other, when such dramatic historical change cleaves apart your respective presents—your experiences of time, your aspirations, desires, and ethical projects? How to build the future that you desire from small, and often banal, acts of presence? How to *continue* to make yourself present to intimate others, even when they refuse, or are unable, to acknowledge the banality of your own present? We saw how elderly women sought acknowledgment of their present through the kind of vital *kaam* (work) that they saw as life-affirming—in the fields, on the shepherding route—even when it was no longer productive. In this chapter I show how younger women also seek this acknowledgment of their present, but through a different kind of labor—the aesthetic and ritual labor of the home. I examine the instances where such acknowledgment is frustrated by economic insecurity and relational conflict, causing the present to become distorted and looping. Drawing on the encounters I had with a number of women across caste groups

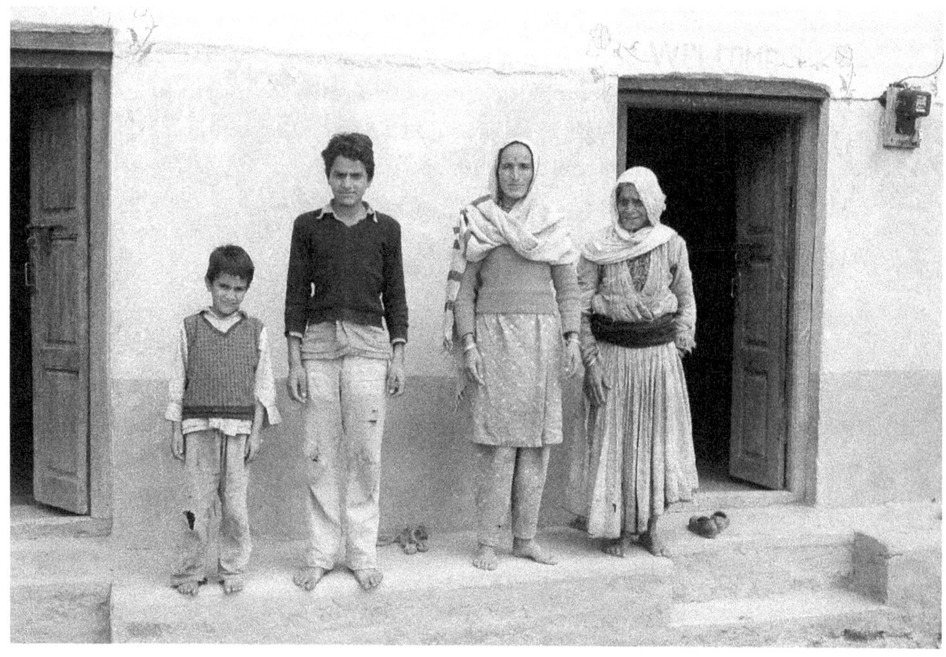

FIGURE 3.2. A multigenerational Gaddi family stands in front of their mud house. The elder grandmother wears the traditional Gaddi *luanchiri*. Note the English "welcome" sign. Today the younger generation of the family live in a concrete house, while the elders still live in this house. Photograph by Peter Phillimore, 1987.

in Thera and surrounding villages, I show how *ghar ki tension* is the experience of this looping present, as it erupts in women's bodies and their homes.

The Housewife

Behind Panchlo's house is a path that leads away from the road toward the fields. Follow it around the galgal tree and through the corn patch, and you reach a lacquered iron gate. Open the gate, and you enter a courtyard, paved with shining slates and lined with potted plants. Cross the courtyard and you reach a house—two stories, painted a pale shade of peach, lined with white cornicing, like a birthday cake. This house belongs to Sapna, Panchlo's *jhetani*, or younger sister-in-law. Unlike Panchlo's house, this house is perfectly rendered. It has none of the overgrown lantana weeds that have now sprung up in Panchlo's beds. It has none of the chipping asbestos or flowering mold that cover Panchlo's second story, worsening after each monsoon.

Sapna was stocky, with a broad, well-made-up face and long hair anointed with vermilion in the parting. While her husband was away, posted with his army regiment to Kashmir or Manipur, Sapna stayed at home. "I'm a housewife," she told me cheerfully when I visited her, sitting in that courtyard surrounded by fields. Sapna's natal home is in a popular tourist spot. She told me this proudly, shooting me a knowing glance that said, "This place is so different, so 'backward.'" She told me that a normal day for her revolves mainly around cleaning and caring for her three young children. She makes their tiffin, a careful combination of healthy vegetables and packaged sweet snacks. She sends them to school, and then she sweeps the floors and folds the bedclothes. She sits down to eat a small breakfast while she scrolls through Facebook, before walking over to her mother-in-law's room to do the same, to administer her medication, and to massage her feet. After an hour of chatter, Sapna returns to the kitchen to make the midday meal. She and her mother-in-law get on very well, but Sapna prefers to keep to herself and doesn't involve herself too much in the goings-on of Panchlo's family or that of her other *devrani*, Anita—the wife of her husband's middle brother.

"This takes my whole day." She smiled.

"And you watch TV," her young son chimed in.

"And TV." She laughed. Sapna especially loves to watch reruns of *Woh Rehne Waali Mehlon Ki*, a popular Hindi serial. Its protagonist, Rani Mittal, is also a housewife—one from a rich family, who gets married into a poor family and learns the struggles of life on the precipice of poverty.

Sapna proudly told me that she doesn't have *tension* like the women of this village. She lamented how tough it was for most women in Thera—those who didn't have the love, and income, of a "good husband." "Gents drink a lot here," she said. "Women have to cope with all of these problems. Where men don't drink, like in my house, they don't lay a hand on ladies. In this place, women aren't strong and assertive. . . . People here talk a lot, particularly about women. People in this place aren't open-minded."

To be a housewife is a relatively new occupation for Gaddi women, just as to build a single, fixed house is a new practice for this previously seminomadic community. However, the house has always been a privileged site for the articulation of Gaddiness, especially for women. In the pastoral economy, men established their connection to the landscape through pastoral labor. Women did so through the transmission of sacred connection to emplaced *kul devis*—clan-based goddesses who reside in houses—and the shared substance of the female line.[2]

The Gaddi house is understood not as a building but as a whole place, where women are said not to have married a particular man but to have married in "such and such a place" and to take on the qualities of that place.[3] Gaddi houses were traditionally made of mud, displaying a unique form of craftsmanship: bricks of earth, dug up and shaped into two squat stories, with low doorways and wooden shutters carved with intricate designs. The interior of the mud house was musty and damp—not with the blooming mold that plagues new concrete houses but with the earthy smell of the dung paint used to plaster the floor and walls and routinely reapplied by the women of the house. Elderly Gaddis described the role of women as "keepers" of the house within the shepherding lifestyle: While men were on the move, women tended to multiple houses along the grazing route. Women were considered equal contributors to the household income. In summer they engaged in subsistence agriculture on the land that their families owned. They supported their husbands with the flock along the pastoral route. And in winter they labored in the fields of landowners in the plains in exchange for lodging and board. Men were often away for long periods, leaving women to manage domestic decisions and care for household gods. Respectability within this role did not depend on women maintaining chastity, such that extramarital affairs and divorce were less stigmatized.

As the agropastoral economy has broken down over the past century, the Gaddi *ghar* has come to be defined by the fixity and boundedness of middle-class domesticity rather than the fluidity of transhumance. Where pastoralism required the pooling of household resources, waged labor requires a division of productive and reproductive labor. Where men are responsible for generating monetary income, women are responsible for small-scale subsistence agriculture and reproductive labor that is framed increasingly as housework (*ghar ka kaam*). This gendered division of labor has been codified in new patriarchal ideals of *izzat*—sexual propriety and respectability. As Kriti Kapila has argued, *izzat* is buttressed by colonial and postcolonial legal regimes of marriage, inheritance, and land registry that shored up the boundaries of the household, specified its makeup, and prevented "improper" practices of polygamy, divorce, and remarriage.[4] Men have seen their dominance over property cemented through the codification of the single male descent line as the primary line of inheritance. Women have seen their right to access or seek maintenance from acquired property diminish, unless it was linked to this ancestral descent line. Families have become nuclear: defined by blood rather than care.

Today the timescape of the Gaddi house is marked by financial flows of wages, receipt of government gas cylinders or below-poverty-line rations, debt repayments, construction work, and the educational cycles of school or college. The house itself remains permeable to the intrusion of playing children;

sadhus (renouncers) demanding alms; salesmen hawking fish, plastic goods, and household cleaning products; and, most important, visiting relatives.

Increasingly nuclear in kinship structure, the household is sustained by a permanent conjugal bond and rigid ideal division between the man as breadwinner and the woman as housewife. For married women, this ability to stay at home and invest in the aesthetics and poetics of homemaking has allowed them to participate in the productive, fertile time of the nation. It was bound up particularly with the performance of a particular sexual chastity that mimics upper-caste respectability.[5] As historians have shown, postindependence middle-class discourse in India sexually objectified tribal women and ascribed to them a sexual freedom that was considered improper for nontribal women.[6] This association between tribal women and sexuality persists today, such that the embrace of lifelong marriage and conjugality is an inherent part of the female role in a collective aspirational pursuit of Indigenous dignity and upward mobility.[7] This is not a straightforward process that mimics Sanskritization for tribal women but a more everyday labor of interweaving multiple projects of self-cultivation that seek both inclusion in a national imaginary and a distinctive place within it.

The materiality of the home—the labor of construction, renovation, and repair but also of cleanliness and curation of domestic space and objects—worked as a sign of this upward mobility. Concrete provided a sign of wealth and displayed the enduring strength of the lineage, while home improvements offered an opportunity to assert wealth and visibility in the community. Women made up for houses that were made wholly or partly of mud with prolific cleaning and populated their interiors with appliances and decorative objects that signaled middle-class status.

Wealthier concrete houses were populated with new appliances, ornate velvet furnishings, and plush blankets, often given as part of a new bride's dowry. In poorer houses, hand-embroidered cushions were laid out on plastic chairs. I was always struck by the immense dignity women drew from these objects. They are largely the same in each place: cream doilies, plastic flowers, studio family photos.[8] Women were keen for me to see these objects, arranging them or showing them to me while we drank tea. In almost every household, I was led to the corner of a room and told to sit on a small couch draped in ornate cloth. The table in front of me was almost always adorned with a plastic vase full of bright fake lilies that sat atop a doily or tablecloth. The peeling walls were covered with garlanded photographs of ancestors or posters of Bollywood heroes. "The composition reminded me of a Deana Lawson photograph," I wrote in my field notes after visiting a Hali woman, who recounted her husband's recent hospitalization in the local psychiatric unit.[9] She served me tea in her best cups, kept only for guests.

Indeed, most Gaddi women were acutely concerned with the cleanliness of their homes. For them, the work of cleanliness involved managing both the vital materiality of the home and of those within it and also a potent immateriality or domestic mood.[10] The aesthetic ideology of Hindu middle-class cleanliness involves the performance of daily rituals to establish boundaries around home and body that exclude the dangerous gazes, bodily fluids, and malign supernatural influences of people considered to be polluting.[11] These might be people from lower castes or classes or those considered sexually unchaste. Cleanliness also involves the management of bodily humors and tempers, for bathing, nutrition, and hygiene promote both physical and metaphysical health.[12] Daily practices of household management, especially in cooking and feeding, are critical aspects of upward social mobility.[13] Gaddi women check food, anoint their children with *kajal* (kohl), and conduct daily protective rituals and prayers to ward off the evil eye. They disallow particular people from entering, sharing food in, or gazing into the home—such as people from lower castes, traveling salesmen, children, women or girls who were considered sexually promiscuous, and even kin whom they believed to be jealous of their wealth. They also manage the boundaries of their own bodies—veiling, wearing appropriate clothing, and, in the case of married women, marking the hair part with vermilion.

This ritual labor has taken on new meaning as Gaddi people have been folded into projects of nationalism in recent decades, and into a turn to Hindu nationalist politics in the present. Like many Gaddi women, Sapna directs daily ritual prayers to Lord Shiva rather than to the family's ancestral god. She participates in contemporary Hindu rituals like *karwa chauth* (a day of fasting for husbands) that were never observed by older generations. Such ritual practice is part of a wider Gaddi turn away from Shaivite animism and toward mainstream Hindu religion, buttressed by the politics of Hindutva. New generations of tribal groups resist nationalist discourses that frame them as "fallen Hindus" by distancing themselves from stigmatized practices such as meat eating, alcohol consumption, and ritual sacrifice.[14] Women have a particular part to play in this project of socioreligious reform. They enter into the masculinist environment of Hindutva through the roles of the heroic mother, the chaste wife, or the celibate warrior.[15] In Gaddi domesticity, these first two ideals combine as the woman's body becomes a site of national and familial honor, her chastity and virtuosity becoming the condition of both familial *and* national thriving.

One male interlocutor explained, "People used to come to India and see poverty in the streets. Now they see wealth and opportunity. They all want to come here. Soon we will overtake those people in the West. They don't even have wives who will have children, so they won't be able to reproduce themselves." As Megan Moodie puts it, "For women who have been excluded from national images of femininity, [d]omesticity is a marker of freedom . . . not a cage from which one must seek release, but a space of security and freedom from worry."[16] Care for a clean home and a sexually chaste, hygienic body are means by which women make claims to upward social mobility and inclusion in a Hindu nationalist imaginary. For many, the value and dignity Gaddi women experience in housewifery seems to refuse the capitalist devaluation of domestic work or the framing of such work as drudgery. As such, Hindutva entered the everyday Gaddi domestic world not through electoral politics but through the inscription of sacred meaning into everyday acts of care (cleaning the body, marking it and dressing it, cooking vegetarian foods, avoiding alcohol, performing acts of fasting) and through the mediascape that women engaged in (the mythical television shows they watched, the WhatsApp messages they shared).

However, as Felicity Aulino has argued, care cannot be tied uniformly to ethical intentionality or an emotional state. Aulino encourages us to think about care as ritual—repetitive acts that achieve effects through their correct performance—in order to attend to what people do rather than what they say they do.[17] I want to take Aulino's argument a step further and attend also to what people *feel* from acts of care rather than what they say they feel. As we will see, the emotions and affects that issue from such repetitive acts of care are not always positive. They are deeply ambivalent, and it is from such ambivalence that distress emerges.

The Web of *Maya*

My favorite time of day in Thera was the hour before dusk. It was a pause in the rhythms of care, between children's homework and the whistle of the first pressure cookers that signaled the evening meal. This was also the time when the sun's last rays lit the peaks of the Dhaula Dhar: pink, orange, gray-blue. Often this lasted only thirty or forty minutes before twilight set in. This was the time for women to go visiting. Some were coming home from their "duties"—their jobs working as cooks, cleaners, or shopkeepers—*sindoor* (vermilion) a little faded, handbags tucked under their arms, pacing rhythmically up the hills. Others emerged from their houses after a day of housework.

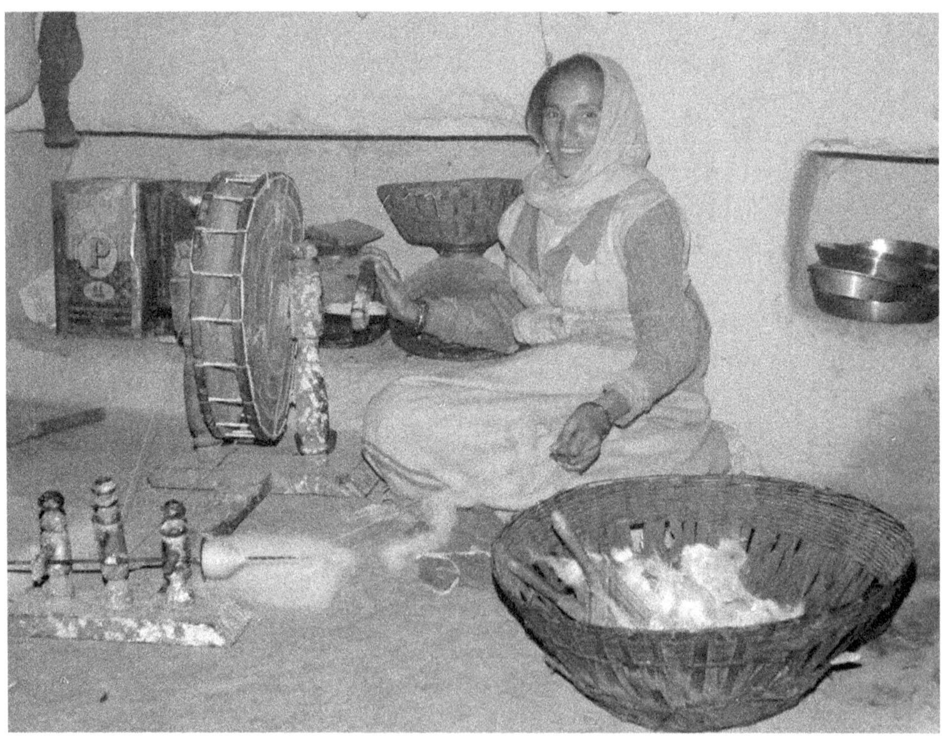

FIGURE 3.3. A Gaddi woman wearing a heavy woolen winter *luanchiri* made by her own hand is spinning wool in her kitchen—an activity that is rare today in Gaddi households. Photograph by Peter Phillimore, 1977.

They sent their children along to the water taps with empty Thums Up bottles and crossed the fields to meet neighbors or sisters-in-law. This was a time to chat, to complain, to joke, and most of all to discuss bodily aches and pains. Do you still have fever? Are your legs still paining you? Have you taken your medicine? Have you rested? *Aacha khana kilaya?* Have you eaten fruits, drunk milk?

In these fleeting moments, the body became the medium of sociality. Women knew that they needed to "share their *tension*" (share *karna parega*), lest the *tension* send them *pagal* (mad). However, opportunities such as these evening exchanges were brief, for women feared sharing too much. They also knew that others had their own responsibilities, their own *tension*.

"Apne ghar, apne tension." (To each their house, to each their *tension*.) This phrase was used to highlight the ubiquity of *tension* in all households. It points to the necessity of keeping one's *tension* away from the prying eyes of others. Gossip and rumor worked as a powerful force, threatening to permeate the privacy of the household, and were considered a source of witchcraft and black magic. Many women expressed an overwhelming sense of isolation and loneliness as new inequalities in wealth between households worked to atomize them and increase suspicion. Those who didn't have financially supportive husbands, especially widows, experienced this most extremely.

It was during one of these evenings that I first heard someone speak about their *tension* as the burden of *maya*. I was sitting with Manju on the roof of her house. We were exhausted after spending the afternoon packing the threshed wheat from her vast fields into large sacks of grain. Manju needed help, for she was a widow. It was a year after the death of her husband in a motorcycle accident, and she complained to me that she experienced both grief from the loss of her husband and anxiety about bringing up her young son without him. I asked her if she had enough support from her sisters-in-law or from her own siblings.

"Zindagi ka saaf koi nahin karte" (There is nobody else who will keep life clean), she retorted as she continued the menial work of packing. She used cleanliness here to refer to the materiality of her home and to the relationships within it.

She continued, "Everybody has their own things. . . . They have to keep their own families. . . . The biggest thing is that you have to think about your own life, you have to think about your own children's lives. Beyond that it is difficult. You have to have the money for your own children's education." Manju's focus had been sending her son to a private school. She had to ask her brother-in-law for the fees and was considering getting a job, but this would cause her to lose respectability in the eyes of her neighbors. These worries, she said, affected her body, leaving her depleted and wracked by *tension*. She spoke of this burden as *maya*.

"[Before my husband died], we were always together. We rested together, we did our work together, we ate together, we didn't spend time with anyone else. But now, after he has passed, I am not interested in worldly things. *Sab moh-maya hai* [Everything is illusory]."

IN HINDU AND SIKH cosmology, the term *maya* is used to refer to the relations, substances, and space of the home and to the illusory quality of worldly things and relations. Anthropologists have focused on the former meaning, framing *maya* as indicative of a particular form of gendered, relational personhood generated through acts of care. Analyzing *maya* among Bengali housewives, Sarah Lamb suggests that it is like a web formed by sharing and exchanging bio-moral substances—such as semen, sweat, and blood—through acts such as having sex, touching, living together, sharing food, owning things, and eating the fruits of village soil; and it is sustained materially and affectively through sentiments of love and compassion.[18] These bonds are made and unmade, in turn causing the humors of the body—heat, coolness, and dryness—to shift. The house is the material space where *maya* is held, such that people are, in E. Valentine Daniel's words, "concerned with controlling what substances cross the vulnerable thresholds of their houses and combine not only with their bodily substance but with the substance of their houses."[19] It is through the control of substances in the house and the substances of the woman's body that the purity of a caste group and a lineage is preserved and reproduced.

Gaddi women used *maya* to refer to the webs of relations they were responsible for, and the consubstantiality of their homes and bodies. However, they emphasized not the positive, life-affirming aspects of *maya* but its negative, illusory qualities: the suffering that comes with care work. For a widow like Manju, well-being would involve withdrawal from the web of *maya*. However, her housework responsibilities left her burdened or stuck in illusion. The association of *maya* with illusion has been said to entrench patriarchal ideas of female deficiency, where women's responsibility for *maya* leaves them unable to understand the true shape of reality.[20] However, Gaddi women spoke of the illusory quality of *maya* as a burden that resulted from their labor. They used the notion to mark the mundane sacrifice that they make for their families, and to push back against their responsibilities. In her encounters with Pahari rural women in Uttarakhand, Radhika Govindrajan also notes *maya* being used to indicate the mundane sacrifice made by women in ceaseless labor with animals and in the home. Her interlocutor, Mohini *chachi*, laments the burden of love (*prem*): "What a thing God has made, this love. After a lifetime of doing work for animals [*jaanwaron ka kaam*], you come to feel such *moh-maya* for them that you can't sleep at night thinking of them trembling in the cold. But in the end, we sell or let them loose after they stop giving milk. . . . This greed for milk is a terrible thing. I don't know if God will forgive us for thieving milk from their calves. . . . Maybe that's why we call it *moh-maya*."[21]

Govindrajan notes that such assertions allow women to push back against the naturalization and devaluation of their caring labor and to position it within wider rubrics of the capitalist economy. For Gaddi women, the assertion of such ethical limits was marked on their minds and bodies in *ghar ki tension*. Overexertion causes depletion of vital energy (*shakti*), resulting in exhaustion, distress, or health problems, but through these forms of disruption, people are also able to articulate their sacrifices.

The representation of the relational web of *maya* as illusory holds within it a particular distorted temporality from which this distress emerges. In its ideal form, the temporality of *maya* is structured by the gift—where mutual obligation, giving and receiving care in the household and through the body, drives time. As Clara Han puts it, referring to the acts of borrowing, cooking, and sharing in the barrios of Santiago, "gifts are given in a modality of reciprocity—of mutual obligations that carry a relation forward in time and in which personal intimacies must be shared."[22] When women give the gift of care—to their husbands, children, natal kin, affines, and neighbors—they give part of their bodily vitality in an act of love (*prem*) to both intimate and divine others. The substances of their body are literally given to nourish their kin and the divine household or god. In return, they expect comfort and well-being. From their husbands, in the form of financial support. From their female children, in the form of support in caring labor. From their sons, in the promise of financial support in their old age.

This care ought to be recognized within the broader structures of virtuous Hindu femininity that is rooted in Gaddi respectability and bolstered by Hindutva. But what happens when acts of care are not reciprocated by others? Or when women do not feel that they receive the emotional or affective return from their emotional labor? In these cases, women feel as though their present, their labor, is not acknowledged. In the case of *kamzori*, we see that this unreturned gift of care is structured by a sacrificial logic, where women feel depleted as a result of a generational debt that is not returned. In the case of Gaddi married women, this unreturned gift of care is experienced as a looping present. Women experience *maya* not as a life-affirming relational network but as a sticky web of worries and worldly concerns that leaves them unable to experience the true shape of reality. In this present, time is always running out.

A Timeless Present

Bimla Didi had a history of experiencing extreme distress. Her marriage, to a hotel chef from her own Gaddi Rajput caste, was marked by periods of conflict, of illness, of violence. At these times I would find her sitting in the front room of her father's home, in the village across the river from Thera. Bimla's own house sits below the road between Thera and Dharamsala, where she and her husband have a small concrete building that they share with their three children. It has a spectacular view that looks upward to the full Dhaula Dhar range and catches the dramatic Kangra sunsets in the evening. Bimla loved to have guests, to invite them to share a meal and stay the night together on mats on the floor. But she insisted that she did not host her mother-in-law, who drove her mad with demands. The space was small, only two rooms, a small kitchen, and an attached bathroom outside, but Bimla kept it fastidiously "neat and clean"—she liked to use the English words.

"When it is not clean, I feel very stressed," she told me. Each day she would wash the pots from the night before, cook the morning breakfast meal, and pack a tiffin for her sons. She would do the morning *puja* (ritual prayers). She would sweep the house with a wide palm broom, polish the ornaments, scrape any mold creeping in through corners, beat out blankets, wash and hang her children's clothes. Then she would make lunch if her husband was home. If she was alone, she would eat a small portion of vegetables left over from the night before or cook herself a simple egg that she ate with sweet bread. Her sons would come back on the school bus, and she would play with them and help them with homework until it was time to cook the evening meal. These endless rituals, she told me, were the source of her home's tranquility and her own personal sense of well-being and pride.

"Women's work is very hard," Bimla muttered to me one day when I was helping her to roll out rotis for her husband's meal. "There is no time for yourself." One of Bimla's greatest sources of stress was maintaining household expenses. This involved the resourceful work of stretching small sources of income and the relational work of seeking support from other family members. As Andreas Streinzer observes, these acts of stretching budgets involve a kind of "time-tricking" that housewives engage in as they face the temporal constraints of economic life.[23] Bimla insisted on sending her children to a private daycare and then to a local Catholic private school, despite her husband's meager income from the restaurant. Bimla's husband is *kanjoos* (tight with money). He "will always go out and eat in nice restaurants himself but will never take [Bimla and her sons] out." Bimla was often forced to beg her husband for money or seek small loans from kin or neighbors to pay for basic expenses like her children's schoolbooks. She explained:

> The main worries are about food and about money. How will we get it? All this *tension*, ladies have. Gents don't have *tension* like this. If, in the house, the rations are finished, the gents will say, Don't worry, I'll earn some money, but they don't say where they will earn that money from. They will say that I will give you this money, and you bring the rations. But ladies think, Where will they do that from? If ladies need twenty rupees, their husband will only give them ten rupees and say, Just make

do with that. Men say, Get the rest of the things later. Ladies say, How will I manage with only ten rupees? Those things are important and are needed right now. Ladies have to adjust.

Women also bore the brunt of any adverse life events like medical expenses, because they were seen as responsible for their household. Bimla Didi explained that she couldn't get the basic checkup she needed from the private hospital because her husband wouldn't pay for it. "2,500 rupees," she cried, "he will start to shout and tell me that I don't have any pain. Women have no time for pain, not body pain or pain in the mind. But when it comes to his costs, like he wants to buy a car, he will just spend the money."

It was of crucial importance that women stopped fights in the home and dealt with domestic violence themselves so as not to disturb the *mahaul* (atmosphere) of the household. Bimla's husband was not violent, but when he came home from a night of drinking, he was often rowdy. He would expect hot, freshly made roti to be served with his meal, whatever time of the night he returned. He would complain that she had not cooked the food he wanted or that it was cold by the time he got to it. Bimla was always worried that he would wake up their two sons, yet she saw it as her responsibility to satiate him, at least for the sake of her children.

Bimla and other women expressed their need to preserve the household temporally, representing their housework as a time loop. They listed their unchanging daily responsibilities, their simultaneous exhaustion and boredom, and the fact that they never had time for themselves. "You don't have the time to go to others' places, to come and go; you have to stay in your own house, eat your own food. You are busy with your own time; you don't have time for anything else, for anyone else. If someone from the road says something bad, then you just have to keep going with your own work. You make your own food, you stay busy. This is what it's like."

We see the Gaddi housewife engaged in an eternal present of care, whereby she must maintain the web of *maya,* remaining constantly present to the needs of others. In doing so, her own sense of time, her own present, dissolves. She has no time. Her present is timeless—both in the sense that she has no time for herself and that there is no end to her caring labor. It is precisely the concealment of eternal labor done by the housewife in the present that allows men, old and young, to engage in leisure time.[24] But sometimes the strains of the eternal present could not be concealed. They erupted into the body as *ghar ki tension*.

Overheated Bodies

I was visiting my family in Chandigarh when I got the call. "Bimla Didi is in the hospital," Shankar blurted out as soon as I picked up the phone. He explained that Bimla had been rushed to the accident and emergency room in the middle of the previous night. As Bimla's second cousin, Shankar got the news quickly from his own mother. The previous day, Bimla had gone to her mother's house complaining of *high BP*. Her head was swimming, and she felt faint. It was only in her natal home, her *maike*, that she would get some respite. Her husband would just have to eat out tonight, she muttered, gritting her teeth against the pain. Bimla had brought her sons with her, and when I had dropped in the previous day, I had played with them on the floor of the living room while she lay on the bed under the fan. Her body was overheating.

When things were particularly precarious, Bimla's *ghar ki tension* developed into bodily symptoms: especially high BP, hot flushes, and acute pains in her body, often in her back or abdomen. She would get a headache and struggle to sleep. These episodes often came after she had had a big fight with her husband. When she felt seriously ill, she would pack up her things and go to her natal home to be cared for. Once she was there, her brothers would take care of her children, and her husband would be left alone to fend for himself. That night her blood pressure got so high that she fainted, and her brother rushed her to the hospital.

IN THESE MOMENTS OF conflict, housework ceases to be life-affirming or a source of dignity for women and instead becomes a struggle. Without acknowledgment or return of their care work, the looping repetition of the present becomes too much to bear. The domestic mood is suffused with *ghar ki tension*. They experience this in their bodies, most often in humoral overheating: when the body and the atmosphere of a house become too hot as a result of relational strain. Heat has been shown by anthropologists of material culture to be an important sensory quality, generated through domestic activities and associated with security and solidarity.[25]

In Hindu cosmology, heat is a particularly important quality of the woman's body, as it is associated with the creative, sexual energy (*shakti*) that is the life force of the household and perpetuates the lineage.[26] At liminal points in a woman's life course, like puberty, marriage, and childbirth, and during breastfeeding, her body is considered overheated and thus the "weak point" in the lineage, where she might invite curses into the household that can afflict her husband

and in-laws.[27] In expressions of *ghar ki tension*, women's bodies would become overheated outside of these liminal junctures as a result of exhaustion or neglect.

Women experienced this overheating through biomedical symptoms like hot flushes, chronic headaches, and *high* BP. *High* BP, though not necessarily medically diagnosed as hypertension, was experienced as an excess of heat that could lead to panic attacks (*ghabrahat*) or heart palpitations (*dil ka ghabrahat*).[28] The sensory qualities of body and domestic spaces caused women to reflect on and resist the expectations of respectability placed on them.[29] Gaddi men lamented that women whose bodies were too hot were impulsive and prone to sexual deviance.

In contrast, women used idioms of overheating to push back against domestic duties. For women like Bimla and Panchlo who experienced these symptoms, the heat of the body marked the overexertion of their energy (*shakti*) and exploitation of their labor rather than its deviant extension beyond patriarchal structures. When the materiality and relations of the household are unbalanced, the very source of life in the house that emits from the female body becomes excessive and tends toward its opposite. The heat of the woman's body that is meant to nourish becomes strange and painful. In these instances, the interiority of the body is overheated and unsettling, just as the interiority of the house is fraught and tense.

WHEN THEY EXPERIENCED *GHAR ki tension*, they could stop working, stop caring. They could seek care from others. *Ghar ki tension* suspended the looping present of domestic labor and brought some kind of respite. However, women were adamant that the temporal break that these erupting sensations brought was not intentional or functional. Nor was the experience of *ghar ki tension* desirable. *Ghar ki tension* was painful, because it signaled a gap between the fantasy of the housewife (the ideal of the home—or *maya*) and the experience of that fantasy itself. Here, the emotions and affects that *ought* to issue from women's caring labor—respect, love, well-being—are absent, and women instead experience shame, fear, exhaustion, and ultimately distress. However, holding on to the fantasy, remaining connected to the ideal of middle-class respectability, necessitates the repression of these emotions. They are encountered only at the edges of consciousness, and they erupt into the body as sensations of overheating, high blood pressure, and other unsettling visceral experiences.

Tine Gammeltoft has charted a similar process by which Vietnamese women attempt to hold on to the fantasy of the happy family that affords them a place in national imaginaries of belonging, despite their experiences of domestic violence. They do this, she argues, by staying silent about their own distress, for to speak would be to kill the fantasy. In Gammeltoft's theorization, the silence itself is an imaginal realm through which these women build images of themselves, interpreting and responding to the symbolic meanings imposed on them. She writes:

> There seemed to be layers in the women's experiences. There were things that could be put into words and things that could not. Experiences that could be immediately shared and experiences that could not. There were stories—about abuse, hurt, distance, and disappointment—that could be told to trusted individuals, even if they were kept hidden from the community at large; and substories—about deep dependencies and fears of detachment—that were more difficult to articulate. Rather than in words, these substories seemed to live in bodies; emerging in tears, in tone of voice, in depth of gaze, in silences between words.[30]

Like Gammeltoft's interlocutors, Gaddi women who experienced *ghar ki tension* were also largely silent about the violence of their husbands and the endless exhaustion from their care work. Instead, they experienced these fraught experiences of domesticity consubstantially in the house and body. In doing so, women obliquely pushed back against the patriarchal and religious structures that left them trapped in a looping present, without letting go of the fantasy itself. "It is through oblique imaginary means [that] the symbolic takes hold in even the deepest recesses of the human organism," writes Jacques Lacan.[31] Indeed, for Gaddi women, the ambivalence, or ambivalent attachment to the fantasy of middle-class domesticity, is worked out and worked on in the deepest recesses of their fleshy beings. In other instances, the unsettling force comes from outside, in the form of supernatural beings that enter the home and body. Let us turn to these instances in the final section.

Jungle Raja Dreaming

Rani was being visited by the Jungle Raja. He came swiftly, in her dreams, tall as a fir tree but stealthy as a mountain lion. At first, he came only every now and then, on nights when she was feeling particularly exhausted. But recently, she told me when we met in Bimla's house over a cup of tea, he had been visiting every night.

Rani was a Hali woman married to a slate miner who was a good friend of Bimla's husband. Bimla had told me before that Rani had been experiencing *ghar ki tension* because her husband's job was unstable, and sometimes he didn't bring home enough money to feed their children. Rani and her husband had been fighting about this, causing the *mahaul* of the house to become fraught. Initially, Rani's blood pressure began to fluctuate. It would get low, and she would become pale and weak, fainting as she went to collect the water or carry loads of grass for their cow. Then it would suddenly skyrocket, and she would become shaky, her hands would tremble, and her breath would get caught in her throat. She came over to Bimla's place when things got too much.

That afternoon, she told us of her visits from the Jungle Raja, also referred to as the Jungle Prince, or the Paharo Walla Raja. He was an incubus that came into the dreams of those experiencing the kind of distress intimately related to sexuality. Most commonly, he came to women who were experiencing *tension* to tempt them into sexual forays. They described him as a handsome man who flattered them before luring them into a forest. Rani explained that the Jungle Raja must be the figure who was also causing other troubles in her life, like her *high BP* and her children not doing well at school.

When Rani went home that afternoon, Bimla explained that she thought the Jungle Raja was visiting Rani because her sexual relationship with her husband wasn't going well, and her husband wasn't earning enough. Bimla noted that Rani's husband had become more attentive since the visit of the Jungle Raja, taking time off to spend with her at home and taking her to a local ritual healer (*cela*).

THE APPEARANCE OF THE Jungle Raja gives us a clue to the significance of sexuality and desire to the condition of *ghar ki tension* and to the fantasy of domesticity. As has been examined, the Gaddi middle-class household has become increasingly nuclear, oriented around a conjugal bond in which female sexuality is located. Meeta, a neighbor of mine, explained the importance of this bond one evening as we sat on her porch.

"Girls, they get married, and then husband and wife, they have sex, and there is a new kind of feeling that happens. They get together, and then they get used to it."

I asked her what this "different feeling" was.

"After marriage, [sex is] like a routine. It becomes an essential part of your life. If you don't do it, you feel weird. . . . For husband and wife, it keeps them together. If nothing else, it's the sex that keeps them together. In the day you're working hard, but in the evening the husband and wife get together." Gaddi women commonly discussed their desires and needs, and ways to cultivate a romantic sexual relationship. However, many women did not have such success. Their husbands were violent, alcohol dependent, or unable to meet their material needs. For these women, *ghar ki tension* was a means to vent unmet desire and express their sexuality beyond the conjugal bond.

The appearance of the Jungle Raja often occurred simultaneously with other symptoms of the overheated body in moments of conjugal strain. In the same way that biomedical complaints allowed women to articulate disrupted care relations, the dreams of the incubus allowed women to articulate unmet desires and often to elicit care from their husbands. These sexual and material desires are linked, and women's expression of transgressive sexuality is a means to navigate domestic situations with agency.[32]

The visits from the incubus recall accounts of spirit possession, which highlight the fraught agency women conjure through these experiences.[33] Also in a Himalayan setting, Radhika Govindrajan recounts a genre of *baat* (happenings) where women are lured into the forest by lustful bears that pleasure them sexually in ways that their husbands do not. *Bhalu ki baat* (talk of the bear), she argues, "allowed women to mount a radical critique of rigid notions of sexual purity and control that portray sexually curious and voracious women as a stigma to their family and community."[34] Similarly, the genre of Jungle Raja dreams allowed Gaddi women to portray themselves as desirous subjects in a way that served their project of middle-class domestic aspiration, pushing back against a hegemonic narrative of tribal sexuality that saw women's desire as corrosive of domestic well-being.

Importantly, however, in both *ghar ki tension* and Jungle Raja dreaming, this expression of agency was not direct: Women did not directly blame their husbands or kin for bodily or psychic disruption, nor did they directly blame their husbands for their unmet desires. Instead, their symptoms and afflictions worked obliquely to signify their strained care relations as they struggled to maintain domestic well-being and respectability in a precarious context. Such expressions of transgressive sexuality occurred in the imaginal realm of the dream. Douglas Hollan writes, "It is the very density, hallucinatory vividness, and ambiguity of dreams and other forms of imaginal thought, allowing them to hold and express a variety of sometimes contradictory or ambivalent thoughts, feelings, and sensations, that make them attractive and mesmerizing to people at times. Such imaginal forms of thought and communication allow us to know things in different ways, consciously and less than consciously, and to know and not know things at the same time."[35]

The Jungle Raja dreams did not break women's faith in conjugality. Instead, they expressed feelings of neglect and desire that were not contained by the conjugal bond. Ultimately, these dreams deepened the experience of the present by allowing Gaddi women to express and hold its ambivalence. They opened new possibilities for acknowledgment and copresence, from the supernatural being himself and from their husbands and friends.

Failure of Fantasy

Why is care so often distressing? This chapter has argued that care is so often the source of distress because it is marked by the impossibility of inhabiting and acknowledging the present of another. In lieu of possible acknowledgment, return for care is sought in emotions and affects that are themselves structured by fantasies. These fantasies, like the fantasy of Gaddi middle-class respectability, "support and give consistency to reality," in the words of Slavoj Žižek.[36] In other words, fantasies allow people to keep caring, despite drudgery, through exhaustion.

Distress reveals both the salience of these fantasies in shaping the affective landscape of the present, and the failure of fantasies to furnish life with the affects that they espouse, especially in relation to care. However, the experience of distress occurs obliquely, at the edges of consciousness—through imaginative thought like dreams, or visceral experiences—such that one can still hold on to the structuring force of the fantasy. In these articulations, we see not only success or failure to achieve the fantasy but also the failure of the fantasy itself to fully interpolate the subject.

In these moments, "domestic worlds and inner worlds tend to collapse," Tine Gammeltoft and Pauline Oosterhoff write, "household tensions and inner tensions blending into one dense feeling of worry and distress."[37] For Gaddi women, these tensions blend at the level of the body and in the context of a high-stakes project of middle-class domesticity. This chapter has attempted to disentangle these tensions by charting a deep history of Gaddi domesticity, showing how the collective aspiration for inclusion in India's (Hindu) middle class is contingent on the labor of women, especially for marginal groups. It has shown, however, that women do not take on this labor unthinkingly, unfeelingly. Instead, many, and especially those who do not enjoy strong marriages or secure incomes, experience this project as a burden that leaves them exhausted.

The looping of domestic labor renders the present fraught in a way that is different from the experiences of their mothers and grandmothers. The present becomes fraught because of a lack of acknowledgment of care—the need to care for others, without the return of care or the emotions that should issue from such care. In moments of precarity, women experience this burden in their bodies, as forms of overheating, high blood pressure, and other painful ailments. In other moments, and especially where their sexual needs are not being met, their dreams are pervaded by supernatural intruders like the Jungle Raja.

These forms of psychic and bodily affliction are painful and distressing for the women who suffer them, but they also allow them to push back against neglectful husbands and abusive kin. They pause the looping present, allowing women to find a seed of relief in the acknowledgment of supernatural beings and intimate others. The articulation of these concerns, however obliquely, is an act of mediating time: both reproducing the ideal of middle-class domesticity and bending, tricking, and distorting the experience of the present through their bodies and in their dreams. Through this temporal mediation, women lamented the immense pressure of sustaining *maya* and also signaled inadequate conditions of intimacy, care, and provision. As such, they revealed the project of domesticity to be not only fundamental to their happiness but also illusory.

4

Future Tension

WHAT IS IT ABOUT THE FUTURE THAT GENERATES DISTRESS?

The Scam

I was shopping in the Dharamsala city market when Rhea called in a panic. I could barely hear her rasping voice over the traffic. When I finally calmed her enough to hear her story, Rhea explained that someone had called her mobile phone, someone she didn't know. They encouraged her to apply for a job in Delhi at one of India's biggest consumer banks. Rhea, having recently finished school and started a course in business administration, jumped at the chance. This was precisely what she had been desperate for—a chance to repay her family by getting a job. They interviewed her over the phone and asked her to send scans of all her documents and her bank details to a new Gmail account. She followed the instructions vigilantly.

A few days later, they called to notify her that she had been accepted for the position. She should be ready to make her way to Delhi the next month,

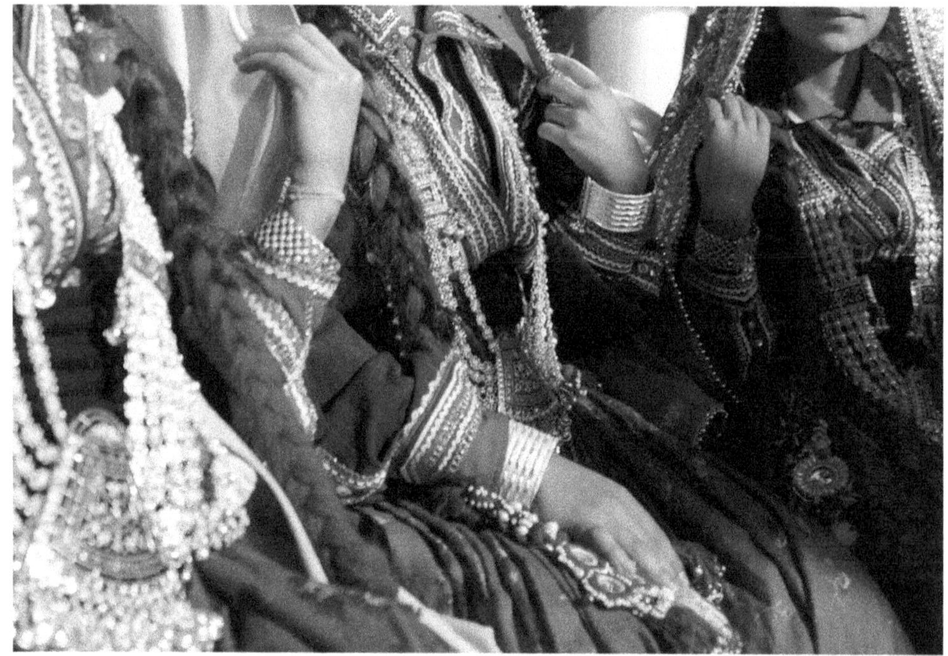

FIGURE 4.1. Three young Gaddi women are dressed in *luanchiri*. Today they wear such traditional dress only at weddings and cultural events. Photograph by Soujanyaa Boruah, 2024.

but first she needed to pay five thousand rupees in uniform fees to a PAYTM account. She asked her mother for the money, and they wired it immediately. This was five days ago, and she hadn't heard from them since. She called the number she had been given repeatedly and sent a deluge of emails to the Gmail account—to no response. When I tentatively explained that I thought she had been scammed, Rhea did not reply.

I met Rhea at a workshop that I ran with adolescent girls of Thera. Afterward, she lingered behind and tapped me on the shoulder. She explained that her family was struggling, and she needed to take responsibility for them. Rhea's father was a Rajput slate miner. She told me he was also a drunk who had abused her mother for years. He had recently left the family for another woman and refused to give her mother any money. Rhea described her mother as a "simple" woman who was uneducated and spent most of her time tending to her cows and small fields. She had no way of making money for the family. Rhea's mother refused to believe that her husband wasn't coming back. To add to this, Rhea's brother was useless, addicted to smoking marijuana and always off on his motorbike. Rhea's sister was meant to get married soon; her engagement was fixed, but the marriage could not go ahead until they had enough money for the dowry payments. Rhea told me that the *bojh* (pressure) was placed on her because she had completed high school and had begun the business course at a private college in Dharamsala. Her father had paid for this and now expected her to start making money for the family. Rhea repeated to me how she had to help her family, support her mother, and bring her father back. She had to make enough for her sister's dowry and indeed for her own, for she owed it to them—they had given her the money for her education, and now she was "just sitting at home" doing household chores.

Rhea wanted a job "like those women who dress up in Western clothes." When I tried to probe about what kind of job she wanted, she only repeated that she wanted to have a desk and a computer but not to have to come home too late. Rhea had no guidance or support from her parents or her siblings. She explained that this burden gave her so much *future tension* that she was always thinking, ruminating, the ideas going around and around in her mind until she felt dizzy. Her body ached, and she felt like she had *high BP*. She explained that she was getting thinner and paler but that if she got her career right, it would all get better. Rhea just repeated, again and again, that she had so much *future tension*. It was making her sick.

MANY YOUNG WOMEN PREFACED their complaints of *tension* with the word *future*. *Future tension* involved excessive rumination, insomnia, and overwhelming feelings of guilt. Girls were also commonly affected by "blood problems"—their "overheated" blood resulted in dizziness, acute abdominal pain, and abnormal vaginal discharge that they called *pani ki problem*. When afflicted by *future tension*, young women's bodies became more vulnerable to *opara* (black magic). In the worst cases, girls were struck down with random seizures, spirit possession, wanton violence, or *dant band*—where they would drop to the floor and clench their teeth until they had to be prized apart by a crowbar.[1] Another friend, Prithi, explained, "Teenagers are more vulnerable to these kinds of attacks of *future tension*. They are not protected, and they don't understand. In their body they feel weak, and their muscles and joints ache, they don't sleep, they don't speak to other people, everything in their lives is *minus minus* [negative]. They go to the doctor because they have *tension*, but the doctors are confused because there is nothing wrong with them. So they go to the *cela* [ritual healer], and sometimes it works, sometimes it doesn't."

For many young girls, *future tension* seemed to bubble up, first slowly, then all at once, at times when a future that they hoped to reach, that they yearned for, seemed impossible or fragile. Their expressions of *tension* seemed to focus on this peculiar experience of time as stretched, fractured, or split between a fraught present and a future shimmering on the horizon.

Gaddi girls were always talking about the future. They most often used the English word but also referred to it as *anevale times*—literally "the times that are coming." These conversations centered on employment, education, and marriage and were performed in the subjunctive mood: "If I could just go on to college in Dharamsala or Chandigarh or Delhi"; "I wish I could find a job in a private company as a receptionist or clerk"; "I hope I find a match, a good boy to take care of me and my parents in marriage."

The orientation toward the future in these conversations was sometimes full of anticipation—joy and excitement for the times to come. Herein, the future shot out from the present, a route that led outward from Thera toward a shimmering, hopeful horizon. At other times, the orientation toward this future was more urgent—the claustrophobia of the present felt unlivable, the stakes of moving beyond that present were high, and women yearned for the future with desperation. At these times, the route to the future did not seem so clear. It was aporetic, leaving women lurching along a foggy road toward something whose shape they could not quite make out. It was in these instances that young women experienced and expressed *future tension*.

The notion of an open future was seen as new for women in the Gaddi community. Elderly women saw their granddaughters as enjoying a great sense of agency to shape and choose their future. The advent of government-mandated education for young people has created a new stage of life, especially for young women, between childhood and marriage. Their grandmothers married soon after their first bleed, or even grew up in their husbands' homes after being betrothed in childhood. As such, they felt little intimacy with their birth families. Their mothers may have been educated until they were twelve years old, unless they were pulled out of school to help with the housework or in the fields. For this new generation, marriage does not come until twenty, or even twenty-four, leaving them free to study until the age of eighteen and even to go to college or get a job after they graduate.

Boys experience great freedom in this time—to use their smartphones, to roam the village, to do *time-pass*, as Craig Jeffrey has explored.[2] Gaddi young men did not encounter the same pressures at this stage in the life course. Boys and young men were concerned with seeking small business loans to open trekking, paragliding, or café ventures; getting government jobs (*naukri*) or enlisting in the military; or pursuing waged employment in the businesses of their kin or in cities like Delhi, Goa, or Dubai. It was important to honor the expectations of their fathers, though they often could not enlist in the same forms of employment in the obsolete shepherding or slate mining economies. This brought distress to young men who were unable to realize both upward class mobility and the distinctive Gaddi *dharam* (moral way of life). However, the articulation and reception of young men's distress, and indeed the sense of futurity that propelled it, was qualitatively different from that which Gaddi girls experienced. Girls, by contrast, are met with heavier expectations to do housework *and* to bring in an income while they still live with their parents. They are encouraged to control their bodily motility and maintain sexual propriety so as to get a good match. Their failures to do so had much more acute effects for the respectability of their kin.

In this context, the future was a time of potential shimmering on the horizon, but young women had no road map and very little support to get there. As such, the demands and dilemmas of the present seemed to intrude on this future, sometimes slowly eroding its sense of potentiality, and at other times erupting and collapsing and destroying dreams. Like their mothers, young women lived the present through looping expectations of household labor—daily chores and duties that filled hours and slowed time. But as we saw in the previous chapter, for their mothers this labor, though exhausting, was also structured by a robust fantasy of domesticity—sustaining the web of *maya* and leading toward middle-class respectability. Young women had a part to play in this project, but it was not their fantasy. They felt responsible to their natal families, but their labor was in service of a household that they would soon leave. In the meantime, they were seen as a source of risk to their kin—an unmarried daughter reaching sexual maturity was vulnerable to the gaze of others and, in turn, rendered the whole lineage vulnerable. Their moves were surveilled, and expectations of propriety appeared as goading words or thinly veiled threats. So the quality of the present, its shape and size, was different for young women. Its edges blended and frayed into multiple potential futures—some prosperous, others bleak.

This chapter is concerned with portraying the quality of this present for young women and questioning why, for these women and for young women elsewhere, this particular period between childhood and marriage is so often a source of distress. Anthropologists have primarily looked at the period of adolescence in contemporary capitalism, particularly in developing economies, as a time of waithood where time-space is compressed. This waithood, in Vincent Crapanzano's words, is "a sort of holding action—a lingering. (In its extreme forms waiting can lead to paralysis.) In waiting, the present loses its focus in the now. The world in its immediacy slips away; it is derealized."[3]

In India, this present-out-of-focus does characterize the experience of some young people, particularly men whose employment prospects are stymied by stagnating wages and job shortages. However, the experience of waithood is not experienced evenly. As Jocelyn Lim Chua argues, late capitalism's time-space compression is not a universal phenomenon. Some experience the present not in a slow, stymied lingering but sped up, accelerated in quickened desires that lead to a different kind of distress.[4] This distress ultimately results in impulsive choices, like the decision to take one's own life.

This chapter shows how, in *future tension*, young women experience both a slow lingering of waithood and an accelerated present. The source of distress is the fluctuation between the two, where young women must balance multiple temporalities of the present at the level of the body. It examines how this results in an experience of time as split, or fractured—resulting in various unsteady, visceral, and even dissociative experiences. It does this through an attention particularly to the life of Ira—my neighbor, friend, and tutee—and her cousins Vaani and Sonali.

Computer Lessons

Ira wanted computer lessons. But it took a month of coming every day to wash the dishes before she plucked up the courage to ask. My neighbor, Uncle Keshav, had implored me to employ Ira to do some work around my house. Though I didn't really need it, for I was happy to wash my own dishes and clothes, he told me it would help her and her family out in a difficult spot. Ira was Uncle's niece, the daughter of his younger brother. She and her family lived in a mud house in the village across the river from Thera. She was the eldest of five daughters and had recently left her higher education in the local high school.

Ira's father had injured his hand in a slate mining accident and was unable to work. Her mother's meager income from her job as a sexual health worker was stable but not enough to support the family and certainly not enough to save for the five dowries their daughters required. Ira's father had already decided to send their middle daughter, Sanjana, to live with her paternal uncle and his childless wife, even though the whole village knew he was a violent drunk. Things were desperate, and in Uncle Keshav's opinion, it was time Ira started to make good on her education and earn for their family.

Uncle's own daughter, Sonali, ran a small beauty business and did piecework for a local tailor on top of her incessant daily work in the house and fields. She kept her orders neatly in an accounting book, and the click and whir of her sewing machine marked the sleepy afternoons. Her work was halted sometimes by a passing client who came to have her eyebrows threaded. Sonali's beauty skills were exceptional. Some time ago, she was an apprentice at a parlor in the neighboring village, until her father's fears about her having to travel the twenty minutes alone became too much for him. Anyway, her parents needed someone to serve tea now, as they were looking for a bride for Sonali's brother and they had too many visitors. The money Sonali generated from her enterprises was fed back to her father. He told me he had to pay monthly installments against the loan he had taken out to build a new story of the house. Sonali had a role to play in this debt repayment while she was between school and marriage. If Ira's family were only a bit more enterprising, Uncle Keshav told me, they might be able to afford a concrete house like his and get a better match for their daughters.

Ira also saw herself as having a debt to pay—a responsibility to help her mother pay for her younger sisters' schooling, her father's medical expenses, and her own future dowry. She began to come over to my house on Tuesday and Friday mornings. On one of these mornings in April, she came earlier than usual. I was sitting on the veranda with my partner, Hugo, drinking my morning tea, when I saw her coming up the stairs. Her scarf was tied practically around her body, and her *salwar* pants were pulled up to reveal feet stained green by the *lipai* (dung) paint that she had obviously been using to refresh the hearth that morning. Her step seemed slow and tired, but as she looked up to see me sitting on the veranda with the usual setup—a fresh-brewed pot of tea on the table, a cup waiting for her—she cracked a smile.

"Hello, Di," she sang. "Hey, Bro." She put out her hand to high-five Hugo. She instantly seemed more at ease.

"Why do you drink that kind of tea?" she asked, stopping to pick up the pot and peer at it strangely. "You don't boil it?"

I shrugged and told her to taste it. I poured her out a cup and added fresh buffalo milk, just boiled after being dropped off by our neighbor's daughter on her way to school. The milk curdled slightly as it mixed with the hot tea. She peered at the swirling colors and slowly sipped it. She made a face.

"It doesn't have sugar?!"

I smiled, and she followed me into the kitchen to get it. She set the tea down and rolled up her sleeves as I went back outside to continue with my work. After some time Ira swept the last of the dust and dirt out the door with a big low movement of the palm broom and set it aside at the edge of the veranda. She repinned her hair and came to sit next to me on the spare cane stool.

"Di," she asked, "will you teach me some things about the computer?"

Ira explained that she had worked very hard in school and had enjoyed the full days there with her friends. But when she had finished, she was just "*aise*"—"sitting" at home, filling her days with the work her four sisters refused to do. She seemed confused. On one hand, she had too much housework to consider doing anything else, like a college course, but on the other hand, she was bored. She felt the hours sieving through her fingers.

We agreed to begin with typing lessons. After she had finished washing dishes and sweeping the floor on those Tuesdays and Fridays, she would come and sit beside me, pour herself some strange tea, and dollop in three generous spoonfuls of sugar. Then I would pass over my MacBook with a fresh Word document open for her. We began with some question-and-answer time, an interview where I would ask questions aloud, and she would type the answers. She was slow and hesitant when picking up skills like spacing, moving back and forth with the cursor, adding capital letters. She looked frequently back at me for affirmation before gingerly continuing.

Evidently, the computer class at her school, which was meant to be a weekly occurrence, had been a failure. A bright young teacher had lobbied the education board to set up a smart classroom and had succeeded in acquiring four computers and a projector. The school was very proud, painting a big sign above the gate reading "Thera School Smart Classroom and Computer Room." But after some months it became clear that the young teacher only wanted to use the smart classroom achievement as leverage to get a transfer to a better school in town. He promptly left, abandoning the computers and projector to the merciless mold of the monsoon.

Ira and I progressed to writing short paragraphs. She would bring a small notebook to carefully write down the English words she was learning and their Hindi equivalents. I would write the same words down in Hindi as I built my own vocabulary. Sometimes when I was out doing an interview, she would let herself in and use one of the old laptops. She traced the keys out onto a sheet of lined paper in her exercise book, trying to establish the pathways between the high *W* and the low *B*, the lines across from *P* to *R* and back again from *E* to *Y*.

Just after the spring wheat harvest and before the planting of the monsoon corn, I noticed that Ira would stop halfway through her typing and look around to see if I was busy doing my own work. I would avoid catching her eye so I could see what her next move would be. She would swiftly switch to the Safari browser and sign into her Facebook account. I was surprised by how adept she was at flicking screens and closing windows, given her wary movements on Word. I realized that she wanted to go on Facebook to speak with her fiancé. I touched her shoulder and gave a knowing smile.

"Who's that?"

She looked away shyly. She told me in a kind of outpouring of coy phrases how much she liked him, how much she was dying to get married, how much she wanted to leave home to go and live in his newly built concrete house with its three tiled bathrooms, marble kitchen bench, and freshly painted peachy walls.

By the time the cornstalks had grown high with the deluge of the monsoon, her voice had begun to crack a little as she spoke about her pending marriage. She would sigh and put her hand to her head. "I have so much *tension*, Di." Day by day, I would hear a little more of the story. Her troubles seemed to multiply. The guilt and shame of being born a girl to a family still fixated on nurturing boys and sending girls away. Her father's meager employment laboring at a hotel construction site at two hundred rupees a day was lost because of a leg injury, machinery slicing his fingers. The realization that her first fiancé wasn't right and the shame of such a blemish to her future marriage prospects. The long and precarious second engagement she had to endure while she waited for her cousins to marry first. "Itne sare soch, Di"—I have so many thoughts.

She explained how the thoughts and worries whirred around her mind. Before, she would come out to peer over my shoulder at the computer screen and wait for her lesson. Now I had to come into the kitchen, where I found her sitting on the cane stool, staring blankly at her mobile phone.

"When are you leaving, Di?" she asked one day when I found her stopped halfway through washing the breakfast dishes. "What will I do when you go?" I reassured her it would be another year before I even thought about leaving, and even then, we would make sure she was able to continue her lessons with someone else.

One evening she came tramping up the stairs. She had missed her morning duties and seemed unapologetic when she explained that she had a new job. "Di, I'm going to work with my sister for a new couple . . . me and my sister. . . . It'll be the whole day. We earn more money." Hugo and I looked at each other. I wasn't surprised by her news, but I was surprised by the rush of sadness that I had. I felt my lips tighten and my fingers flex.

Investing in Girls

A new generation of educated young Gaddis eschew not only the agropastoralist livelihoods of their grandparents but also the military and *masdoori* (waged labor) in the slate mines or construction industries that their fathers

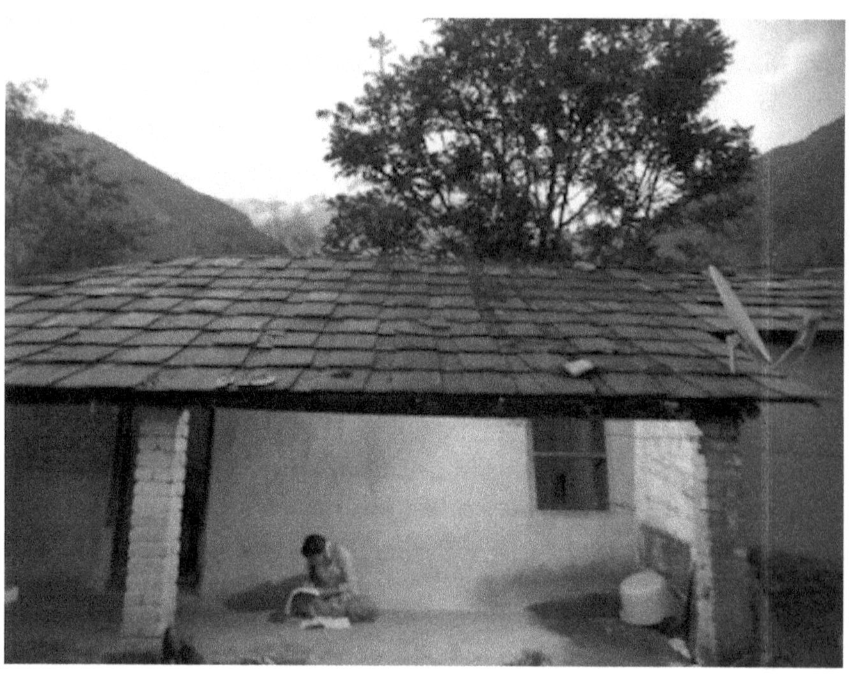

FIGURE 4.2. A girl does her homework before attending to dinner. Photograph by Nikita Kaur Simpson, 2018.

pursued. Young men particularly want *naukri*—government white- or green-collar jobs. More recently, in the wake of liberalization policies that have ramped up in Narendra Modi's India, young men have begun to aspire to be entrepreneurs, taking advantage of loans made cheap by affirmative action benefits, increased tourist demand, and migration opportunities. These are sustained by vast networks of caste-based patronage where young people are supported, often by men like Uncle Keshav who have access to capital and credit as a result of their military pensions. The appeal of new public and private sector livelihoods is not just economic—getting a *naukri* or starting a business is also essential to a good marriage match. However, precisely at the point when young people are taught to be modern at school and college, and their aspirations to middle-class identity intensify, they experience a decline in real opportunities for white- and green-collar employment across India, leading to a culture of aimlessness, particularly among men.[5] Further, the success of microenterprises is often fleeting: The main road in Thera is littered with discarded signs and concrete structures—a graveyard of young men's business dreams that never quite took off.

As such, many fathers told me that "investing" in their daughters was more logical than investing in sons who only wanted to do *time-pass*. Where daughters are likely to care for their parents in old age, even if they move away for marriage, sons don't have the same respect for their families and only go and spend money on their own wives. Parents talk of investing in stitching courses and sewing machines, in computer skills courses and laptops, and providing capital for small enterprises in or close to the home like beauty parlors or boutiques selling hand-stitched kurtas.

Before marriage, girls are expected to pursue education, business, and employment opportunities while staying close to home and continuing to perform their domestic chores. Indeed, marriage was the most durable marking on the temporal horizon for young women like Ira. The will to earn an income is driven by the need to secure a good match for themselves, earn the money for their dowry, and contribute to the dowry of their sisters. The very meaning and shape of marriage has changed for adolescent girls. In the past, girls were promised in childhood and stayed with their natal family until the age of thirteen or fourteen. Then they would be married in *atta-satta*, or exchange marriage within caste groups, without a dowry, and would move to live in their marital home. Their value to their natal family was in their domestic labor, which would have to be replaced when they married. In this context, families lamented that they should not get attached to their daughter as she would only move away—leaving the emotional tie between the daughter and her natal home weak.

However, the past fifty years have seen significant changes in marriage practices—the average age of marriage has increased by a decade. By the 1970s Peter Phillimore observed that most marriages were framed by *dan-pan*, or marriage by gift, a trend that had intensified by the time of Kriti Kapila's research in the early 2000s, when marriages were increasingly framed by mainstream Hindu values. Today the meaning of marriage has been further appropriated as a means of gaining status. Upwardly mobile Gaddi families have adopted hypergamous prestige marriage practices—where marriage becomes an opportunity to increase class status *and* cement caste endogamy.[6] In this context, a dowry becomes—in Veena Oldenberg's terms—"a net" for the natal family to catch a good, high-class suitor and maintain a good lineage.[7] It is also a potential means for the marital family to speculatively extract wealth from the natal family, to control and suppress a new bride. As such, gathering the dowry is a great strain on family resources, and this strain falls on the bride herself.

The benefits of investing in girls could even last beyond their marriage. Where in the past young women were encouraged to cut ties with their natal family when they were married, today advances in transport and social media mean they can visit and care for their families much more often. The tendency to set up a separate concrete house for a son and his new wife, as opposed to setting up only another hearth in the same mud house, weakens the ties between the couple and his parents. Daughters, even if they are married, are called back to care for their aging parents and give money in times of need.

GADDI GIRLS' POSITION IN the Gaddi domestic economy is underwritten by the increased value of the "girl child" in the Indian women's empowerment policy, which filters down through local government and nongovernmental organization (NGO) efforts. For example, the "Beti Bachao, Beti Pradhao" (BBBP)—"Save the Girl-Child, Educate the Girl-Child"—program, launched in 2014, promotes the increased "value" of the "girl-child" in the household through a suite of education, awareness-raising, and financial inclusion policies aimed at preventing sex-selective abortion and encouraging families to send their daughters to school.

One of the most interesting policies is the Sukhaya Samriddhi Yojana, an initiative that encourages families to set up a bank account for their daughters before they are ten, where the family's payments are matched by an 8.5 percent interest rate funded by the government. The account remains open for twenty-one years. Half the money can be withdrawn after the age of eighteen for higher education expenses, and the full amount can be withdrawn by the family when the girl gets married. Critically, this kind of financialized "empowerment" policy is aimed at changing the cultural attitudes of families toward their daughters by increasing their financial value.

These kinds of "invest in the girl" policies are part of a global economic agenda that sees educated girls as yielding a higher rate of return than other forms of investment in the developing world. The shift in the subject of development policy from the worker or consumer to the entrepreneur sees, in Michelle Murphy's words, "'[the] Third World girl' becoming the iconic vessel of human capital. Thoroughly heterosexualized, her rates of return are dependent on her forecasted compliance with expectations to serve family, to adhere to heterosexual propriety, to study hard, to be optimistic, and hence on her ability to be thoroughly 'girled.'"[8] These novel Indian policies see young women as assets to the household not merely for their labor power, like in older policies of NREGA (National Rural Employment Guarantee Act, 2005), for instance, or through the need to directly control her reproductive decisions, like in the early childhood and sexual health programs. Instead, they see the abstract figure of the adolescent girl as an entrepreneurial asset to both the domestic and national economy. This is manifest both in opportunities given by the government to integrate women into the workforce to generate economic value and in the need to put cash into the hands of their household in order to increase its consumption power.

Here we see the young girl's body as a site of potentiality. "Potentiality," Gisa Weszkalnys reflects, "presents itself both as 'futures fold[ed] into presents' . . . and as something stymied, marked by blockages and setbacks."[9] The condition of this potentiality is her compliance with the gendered expectations of her family and community. These policies are aimed not at providing her with decision-making power independent of her family but at increasing her value to the household. Indeed, they exploit the expectation placed on a young woman to remain obedient to the decisions made by her father and to absorb caring labor in the household so that the value she accumulates can be channeled back into the family. The move to invest in daughters is unmatched by a logic of independence, and any idea of women's empowerment is not an assumption of individual flourishing. Instead, as anthropologists studying women's microfinance have found, the very foundation of neoliberal empowerment policy is this gendered, radically relational subject.[10] Young Gaddi women see themselves as implicated in constitutive intimate relations to which they are accountable. Envisaging a future for themselves does not involve cutting themselves off from these networks but finding a way to improve the comfort, security, and well-being of those in both their natal and their future marital homes.

As one young woman told me while we were washing clothes together in the local stream, "There's no such thing as independence. It's more important to have a good husband than to have individual freedom [*azadi*]." I paused, wondering what it was about *azadi* that made it so risky.

Vaani's Excursion

Vaani had been gone for four hours by the time they called me. I had just stacked the dinner dishes in the sink when I heard Sonali shouting for me on the steps. Usually, Uncle Keshav and Sonali were asleep by this time—lights off and doors bolted against the February chill. But today something stirred in the hamlet. I met Sonali on the balcony. "Is Vaani here?" she asked quickly, eyes darting behind us. I hadn't seen Vaani—Sonali and Ira's cousin—since she and the other girls had come over to my house for a movie night a few days before. She regularly dropped in to see me and my housemate after school or in the early evening. She would flash her coquettish smile at Hugo and look at herself in the mirror pinned to our *almirah*. Vaani was one of the "*frank* girls" at school—popular but impulsive. She wore thick black eyeliner on her top lids and never brought her scarf out with her. Sometimes she even wore jeans and sneakers. She also used our home as a sanctuary from her turbulent family. Sonali sighed, knowing even before she asked that Vaani wasn't here, and headed back downstairs to tell her father.

I woke in the morning to shrill shrieking. At this point in my time in the village, I could well identify the shriek as that of Neha, Vaani's mother, who loudly fought with her mother-in-law in their front courtyard. Such shrieking blended into the usual morning sounds of the goat bleating below my bedroom window, and the bells of the cow and her calf being taken to graze. Vaani's house was slightly up the hill from ours, such that from my window I could see it like a raised stage. Through the crack in the curtains, behind layers of apricot and walnut trees, I could see a number of people milling around two women who were clearly pitched against each other. It was Neha and her mother-in-law.

Neha pulled at her thinning hair and appeared to double over as her mother-in-law waved a long stick just above her bowed head. Neha's fraying kurta hung loosely on her slight frame, seeming to skew to one side and baring her shoulder like a boiled hen's egg. Her mother-in-law sneered. Her insults only cut with crueler precision because of Neha's shrieking. Neha's mother-in-law brought the stick down against the slates, missing Neha's feet by centimeters. I could just see Vaani's wide-eyed face. It was as if the scene had been made publicly for the benefit of the neighbors.

I asked what was going on and was told that this fight had gone on all night last night, then started again this morning. They told me that Vaani had gone missing the previous evening. She and two girls from the upper village had gone to a DJ party in the nearby military cantonment without asking her mother's permission. Her father and uncle went to find her. They searched every wedding that was going on in the neighboring villages but returned empty-handed.

It was not until well after midnight that Vaani returned home in an unmarked car with two other girls, driven by an unknown boy. The fight had begun when Neha picked up a long stick used to swat the cow and began lashing out at her mother-in-law and husband for not finding her daughter. Then her mother-in-law grabbed the stick and started to hit Neha, yelling to the whole village that Vaani's behavior only mimicked her mother's. She waved the stick around above her head, and each time it came down a little closer to Vaani, who sat close to the action.

That evening, Shankar and I were huddled in my room around the strip heater when we heard a knock at the door. "Nikitaaaaaa," came Anu's high-pitched nasal voice, making us cringe as she poked her head around the door. "Do you have a broom? I need it to do the floor in the morning." Anu was Vaani's aunt. A thickset lady with a sweet face that had been beautiful when she was younger, before her daughters came—one, two, three, four, five—and the hope of having a boy faded into lines webbing her eyes. Anu knew precisely where the broom was. After the story about Vaani broke, I had expected her to drop by soon. Anu was another woman who often came to our home and loved to share the whispers and rumors of the village. Whenever you met Anu, you were sure to hear of some elder woman who had found a pile of ash in her kitchen pantry, a spell laid by a jealous sister, some young girl run away with her college boyfriend only to return bruised and tattered.

Anu humbly excused herself for disturbing us. She drank in her surroundings, having never been into my room before. Then, satisfied, she crouched down in front of us and promptly forgot the ruse of the broom. It was clear that things had changed since the morning, and the tide had shifted against Vaani—within the space of a day, she had moved from being a victim of violence to a dangerous influence. First, Anu told us exactly what had happened. The incident was clearly an opportunity to open the floodgates against Vaani and her mother. Anu's visit to us was a means of distancing herself from their shameful ways, setting herself and her own daughters safely away from the depths of critique. She paused, inviting us to fill the gaping unaccounted-for period with our dangerous speculation. "There is no knowledge of where she was or what she was doing," she emphasized. Anu's tone changed, and she leaned forward slightly on her haunches. The reason she was telling us was purely, she said, to warn us. And here she paused to allow the sense of danger to fill the space between us. Vaani's behavior was unacceptable. And it had happened because she had been able to come to our home. She warned us not to allow Vaani, or any of the other children, to come to our place, lest we be blamed for facilitating their errant behavior.

After the incident with Vaani, most of the mothers stopped sending their kids out to run from kitchen to kitchen. Women became more suspicious of one another when a woman would come back late in the evening. Even we kept to ourselves more. Just as Ira had used our house as a place of escape from her mundane chores, Vaani had used our house as a place of escape from her family and as an alibi to slip away unnoticed. Indeed, Anu's warning was also a threat. Young women, if left to their own devices, were a source of risk.

Potential, Risk, and Respectability

When Vaani went missing, I was reminded of the first summer I spent in Kangra. It was 2014, and I was twenty-one, in the final summer of my undergraduate degree. I, too, moved through the villages of the Dhaula Dhar saddled with warnings about what happens to girls who stay out too late. It was two years after the Nirbhaya incident in Delhi. Like me, everyone knew the contours of Jyoti Singh's story. How, on a cold December night in 2012, she and her boyfriend had gone to see a movie in South Delhi and boarded an unmarked bus. How she had protested when the bus headed off in a different direction instead of toward her home. How the six men on the bus closed and blocked the doors, knocking her boyfriend down with an iron rod. How they proceeded to gang-rape Singh for the next hour while the bus drove through the streets of South Delhi. How they inserted an iron rod into her vagina, ripping apart her intestines, abdomen, and genitals.

Nirbhaya, in Hindi, means fearless. It was the name given to Singh by the press in the days after her body was found on the side of the road, as she was struggling against the injuries she would ultimately succumb to. Her ravaged body loomed large in the collective imagination of the country that summer as the streets of India's urban cities filled with protesters—some demanding freedom for women in public space, others demanding retribution. In Kangra, stories of Nirbhaya were traded not to show fearlessness but to inspire fear.

"There are thousands of girls like Nirbhaya," a Gaddi community leader contended, "but they didn't go outside of the house after eight. . . . Why did she throw her life away at just twenty-two? If you live with ethics, your life will be long."

"Women should look to Sita as a role model integrated into modern life," a local panchayat member echoed. "She tells us we should not cross boundaries."

"Western ideas of sexuality don't complement our culture," a policewoman reflected. "The mentality is different. We are undergoing transformation, we don't want to give up our values, but we want to be modern. Which culture will we follow?"

When I first began to talk with young women, in that summer of 2014, about what they thought of the Nirbhaya incident, they took a long time to answer.

"That doesn't happen here," they surmised, clearly distinguishing between the safety of the hills and the danger of the city.

"It is *kharab kaam* [bad work]; it is not good for girls and women," they whispered.

"After it happens, if a woman goes outside, she will become shy and never tell us," one young woman, Sarika, told me as we hung bedsheets out to dry.

When I returned in 2017, the sexual panic surrounding Nirbhaya had fermented, leaving in its wake a more mature and muscular discourse surrounding the plight of young women who stepped too far beyond the boundaries of the village. This discourse was repeated countless times, especially by upper-caste elderly Gaddi men who seemed keen to monitor and preserve my own respectability as much as that of their daughters or granddaughters.

I HEARD THIS MOST clearly on a hot June day when I met Suresh. The whole village was talking about one such incident. A young woman was found hanging from a fan in the living room of her new husband's house. This woman was just married, so recently that she still wore red bangles up her forearms. At first, it had been ruled a suicide. Perhaps she had not been able to cope with the demands of marriage, or she hadn't been able to adjust to her new household. But for her mother, and for her friends, this seemed out of character.

The young woman had been accomplished and independent before marriage. She worked in a local NGO and had met and married her husband after months of dating. It was a love marriage, to a man of a different caste. Her family had protested, but the marriage had gone ahead. As the facts of the case became clear, a suicide looked less likely. Rumors began to circulate that this woman was killed by her husband. We can recall the words of Deepak, the elderly Gaddi Brahmin we met in chapter 2: "In the new generation, the [mental] changes that have happened to girls have been caused by the control of society."

Young women, as they become sites of potentiality and investment, also become sites of risk to the lineage that must be controlled. As Sumi Madhok and Shirin Rai argue, "Risk is the inherent danger that dwells in the moments of transgression of these social relations; it disciplines agents and attaches itself to defiant bodies and social spaces where acts of defiance are performed."[11] Culturally, such risk is framed as a young woman's *shakti*—her sexualized power to create or destroy the lineage and its *izzat*. Her *shakti*, contained in her body and especially in its substances of blood and vaginal fluids, must be controlled and domesticated through a learned set of bodily dispositions and skills. These are acquired through both positive engagement and the threat of punishment if the woman innovates too far from the norm.

Changes in Gaddi kinship and marriage systems have worked to amplify the riskiness of the adolescent girl in the present moment. In the past, girls were promised in early childhood, then married when they reached puberty. Today, due to the illegality of child marriage, engagement and marriage rituals are performed within the same period, opening up a stage of adolescence wherein she might go to school and her sexuality must be controlled. During this period the adolescent girl's body is described as hot and open (*khola*). She is vulnerable to the intrusion of the sexualized gaze of men from other communities, as she is to the intrusion of supernatural forces. For this reason, adolescent girls are often the subject of attacks of *opara* and *jadu* (witchcraft). They absorb a curse directed at the whole family, as they are like the "weak spot" in the family's constellation of *izzat*. During this period it is of even greater importance that the adolescent girl's body, movements, and behaviors are controlled and surveilled in order to maintain her chastity.

As Sohini Kar puts it, control over sexuality becomes a means by which the investment in the woman is *securitized*.[12] Adolescent girls are permitted to generate economic value for their families, allowed the freedoms this necessitates, so long as they stay within the terms of the investment, terms securitized by their *izzat*. So we see that an adolescent girl whose family has invested in her education is, first, acutely burdened by the responsibility to channel return from this investment back to her family; and, second, acutely aware of the risk of such endeavors lest she step too far. My interlocutors told me stories of the risk they undertook in working in Dharamsala or traveling to and from college; parents, teachers, and news media blared dramatic stories of girls who went too far—found raped on buses, kidnapped in taxis, abandoned by boyfriends, sold into sex slavery in Goa. Spectacular instances of sexual violence like the Nirbhaya incident, along with local femicides, become the means by which the adolescent girl is framed as a risky subject in the popular imagination, defining the limits of her freedom and the consequences of stepping too far.[13] But the responsibility for managing one's own risky body, while also making good on relational obligations, becomes too much for some.

Ilaaj

Ira first experienced pain in her stomach soon after she stopped working at my house. Still in need of money, she and her sister Shivani went to work for a "foreigner" couple some twenty minutes by bus from our village. The couple ran a home massage parlor that catered to the steady stream of Israeli, European, and American tourists in the area. The sisters were employed from 9 a.m. to 5 p.m. each day, seven days a week, to clean and learn basic skills in massage. It was unclear whether their obligations involved any kind of sex work, but such massage parlors dotted the valley. They were paid sixteen rupees per hour. Their mother had arranged the work for them out of desperation.

"A respectable family would never allow this kind of work," Uncle Keshav tutted, ashamed of his sister-in-law. Ira and Shivani went back and forth on the bus each day for a month; then one week I noticed that they had stopped going. I asked Uncle why they hadn't gone to their job, and he told me that Ira was feeling very sick—she had a sharp stomachache, she felt dizzy, and she was losing weight. Ira had had *tension* before—a looping rumination that stopped her from coming to our weekly computer lessons—when worries about her sister's marriage, her father's injury, and her mother's debts had absorbed her. But this seemed more acute.

First, they had taken Ira to the Zonal Hospital, where she was kept under observation for four days. On day two, Shivani had also been admitted, clutching her own abdomen. After a succession of consultations in the crowded outpatient department, after blood tests and body examinations, they could find nothing clinically wrong with either of the sisters. Their mother tutted and fussed around them. "It's *tension ki bimari*"—*tension* sickness—she told me on the day Ira and Shivani came home from the hospital, shrugging her shoulders. I saw them that day, bundled up on the veranda of their small mud house as onlookers whispered.

"Maybe they feel shame for some kind of physical relation they're having," suggested Asha, a neighbor who worked for a local NGO.

"These girls already go and stay with their fiancés, and maybe the family wants to direct blame away from this so as to keep the engagement fixed," Sukriti, another neighbor, tutted.

Indeed, moments where *tension* erupted out of bodies publicly, as in Ira's case, presented moments of impasse within social relations—"an interruption," in the words of Lauren Berlant, "to the norms of reproductive life that can be adapted to, felt out, and lived."[14] In these moments of impasse, the future seemed to become suspended for the afflicted and was the object of intense speculation for those around them. They became a lightning rod for the skepticism that rippled through everyday life. Too often, these moments ended with an *ilaaj*—a treatment, an act of ritual discipline, or even violence, that worked to manage the unruly girl's body or truncate her future possibilities.

As night fell on Ira's house, a line of relatives had begun to congregate in the courtyard. Two unknown men stood out to me among the relatives—a thin man in spectacles and an old man in tattered trousers. I snuck off back to my own house. Those men, Uncle Keshav told me when I returned, were a *cela* and his assistant. They were here to perform the *ilaaj* for the whole family. Indeed, it was not only Ira and Shivani who had experienced *tension* and other ailments acutely in recent months. Their *tension* seemed to run along the relations of the family. Their aunt had begun to have extreme menstrual pain, and their uncle had begun to have strange episodes of vertigo after falling from a tree. But the *ilaaj* centered on Ira, for it was the *tension* in her body that was emanating out and across the domestic network, threatening the lineage, they said.

Ira's mother spoke of how they needed to remove the *tension*, lest malign spirits enter their homes and take a human sacrifice. The beating of drums began as I was dropping off to sleep that night and didn't stop until dawn three days later. It was on that third day that I found Ira shivering on the stoop. And it was only another three days after the ritual that Ira's pain, and her *tension*, returned. Indeed, the stories of those who experienced *tension* evaded redemptive narratives of recovery or deliverance. For, in most cases as in Ira's case, *tension* might abate, but it could not be cured. Its remedies might bring release, but they did not bring certainty or stability.

That morning after the *ilaaj*, Ira trembled on the stoop outside the kitchen. It was the morning after she had sat face-to-face with the healer; after her hair had come loose from its clasp; after she had been whipped with the *sangal* (whip) until she was exhausted. She stank of smoke when I came to sit beside her. She was waiting to shower in the stall of her uncle's house, for her own house didn't have a toilet, let alone a shower. She let me wrap my arms around her, but it did nothing to calm her shivering.

"Is the pain gone?" I asked, quietly.

She looked up at me. "The stomach pain is gone, Di," she whispered, "but my neck hurts from all the thrashing."

"And the *future tension*, is it still there?"

She fingered the nape of her neck lightly, as if feeling the pain in this new place, how her muscles would have to shift to accommodate it. She folded her head onto her knees and rocked her hips. We sat in silence in the brightness of the May morning. I couldn't tell whether she wanted me there or not, but I felt her *tension*. It moved against my shoulders. Cold, despite the warmth of the ten o'clock sun on my arms. I remember thinking that perhaps I could hold some of it for her, for a moment. Soon her uncle emerged from the shower, combing his mustache. He patted his niece on the head, and she rose.

"She will be OK now," he assured me, and perhaps himself, as she closed the door behind her.

The Future Is in the Present

Future tension is, to riff off Michelle Murphy's words, "both a temporal orientation toward the future and an affective state, an excited forward-looking subjective condition of yearning, desire, aspiration, anxiety, or dread."[15] Without the affective structuring that is provided by a durable fantasy like domesticity, which their mothers pursue, young women experience a sense of deep disorientation in emotion and in time. The potentials imbued in adolescent girls by their families provide new possibilities for imagining a future. Yet, taken together, instances of *future tension* show that this future is stymied and fraught, such that this position holds an embodied cost. This is particularly the case for aspirational girls who are given the responsibility of the whole family's well-being but also must manage their own risky bodies. For those like Ira and Rhea, for whom class and caste status concerns render the stakes the highest, the everyday management of financial, sexual, and moral risk tips into *future tension*. Without a clear way forward, a means of acting on their potential, the future seems to recede into the horizon. While young men also encounter this shimmering horizon, I was told that they don't experience the same kind of *future tension. Future tension* is explicitly gendered because young men's bodies do not hold such relational risk.

The temporal landscape, and the experience of the present for these Gaddi girls, is quite different from the present that is captured in studies of waithood, or the binary present that is represented in the "cultural struggles" of young women who move between their village or family life and other, more modern spaces.[16] Instead, in *future tension*, the pressure of the future collapses into the present. Young women are forced to manage multiple temporalities—of economic and kinship potentiality, of libidinized risk, and of domestic labor. Their temporal orientation to the future thickens the present with ethical dilemmas and unsettling affects that pool in the adolescent girl's body. Managing the riskiness of their bodies requires young women to speculate in order to elicit a radically uncertain future, and to mediate it with a looping domestic present.[17] Such dilemmas are experienced somatically because the symbolic idiom of sexual risk is conceived through ideas of the hot and open adolescent body, vulnerable to penetration by external actors and holding the respectability of the group. The body holds the imagined and experienced weight of household relations at a particular point in the life course. The burden is too much to bear for some, particularly those of lower-caste or lower-class aspirational households for whom the stakes are highest.

In short, young women's bodies experience a splitting or fracturing of time—where the present blends into and even shatters under the weight of the future. The relation between the present and future here is not linear. "But must the future and the present exist in this rigid binary?" asks queer theorist José Esteban Muñoz in his essay "The Future Is in the Present."[18] Muñoz argues that some acts of "performance—both theatrical and quotidian—transport . . . us across symbolic space, inserting us in a coterminous time where we witness new formulations of the present and the future."[19] Muñoz writes of queer communities, of people of color, of "minoritarian" groups, for whom the present is like a cage, and the future is elusive or unwritten. For Muñoz's minoritarian groups, as for the Gaddi young women who experience *future tension*, the present and future are experienced simultaneously, not in binary opposition. This nonbinary relation of the present to the future can be a source of distress.

The experiences of Gaddi women here resonate with a case that the psychotherapist and anthropologist Rebecca Lester discusses: Ella, a client diagnosed with dissociative identity disorder who performed multiple ages at the same time.[20] Lester writes:

> I saw something similar in Ella's experiences of self, in that different parts existed at different times—yet also in the present—and she struggled to form a coherent sense of herself as a result. Ella herself thought of this as what she called a "telescoping process," with parts stretching back across time while also being present in the present day. Parts were therefore not solely located in any one temporal domain but telescoped time. Furthermore, while some parts remained the age the body was when they were made, parts of any age could be created at any time. So, in addition to telescoping time, parts could actively use temporal displacement as part of their communicative function.[21]

For Ella, as for Gaddi women, *future tension* was a dissociative experience whereby time was split or fractured. The experience of mediating multiple temporalities in the body became painful and unsettling, or even unbearable. Lester suggests that the different temporal parts Ella inhabited had communicative functions. Here I depart from her analysis, for I didn't see *future tension* as having a primarily communicative function. Instead, the pains and aches of the condition introduced a pause in social relations whereby multiple temporalities might be felt out and untangled, and where the present might be rendered consistent through acts of care from others. However, these acts of care were also acts of domination, where temporal experience of the body is restructured through ritual time.

Often, episodes of *future tension* ended in rituals similar to the *ilaaj* that Ira was subjected to. In these instances, the resolution to young women's distress is their further integration into domestic structures through ritual exorcism. These rituals are unlike the private one-on-one ritual therapy between an afflicted person and a *cela*, or the public ritual events where deities might become involved in matters of collective political decision-making.[22] Instead, such events are focused on the domestic group—on both articulating social subversion and reinscribing patriarchal, intergenerational, and classed configurations of authority.[23] They work to collectively hold the ambiguities of *future tension* and to disperse its negative effects across the domestic network. On one hand, the complaints of *future tension* illuminate a form of visceral refusal articulated in and through the body. The act of agency on the part of the adolescent girl is a relational one—to articulate the immense pressures of care, risk, and work placed on her; to identify its causes in fraught, particularly domestic, relations; and to push such pressure back onto those relations themselves as a means to seek help. On the other hand, in such moments of crisis, community as a "set of acknowledgements," as Veena Das puts it, colonizes the individual's lifeworld by defining the limits of selfhood, by centering time.[24] Often, the time that is centered is the time of the life course, the next stage of which is marriage. This recentering occurs through the very symbols and metaphors of the ritual exorcism, Isabelle Nabokov argues, whereby women's distress is rewritten according to hegemonic idioms that bolster patriarchal normative structures within the family.[25]

Coda

I heard the singing from the wedding house before I saw it. The sound of the *dhol* (drum) was rhythmic, blocking out the car horns and the calls of the black bulbul. It was four years since I had heard these wedding songs. I followed the singing into the house, sucking in my stomach and putting my hands above my head to squeeze past the many people packed into the small courtyard. I knew the girls would be there. Ira and Sonali certainly would, for it was their cousin's wedding—they would have to come back from their own marital homes to be part of the festivities. I picked my way across the veranda, finding spaces for my feet between lounging and chatting and singing women. They were all dressed in their best silk suits. They wore their own wedding jewelry, their faces obscured by intricate *maang tikka* (head jewelry) that hung on their foreheads

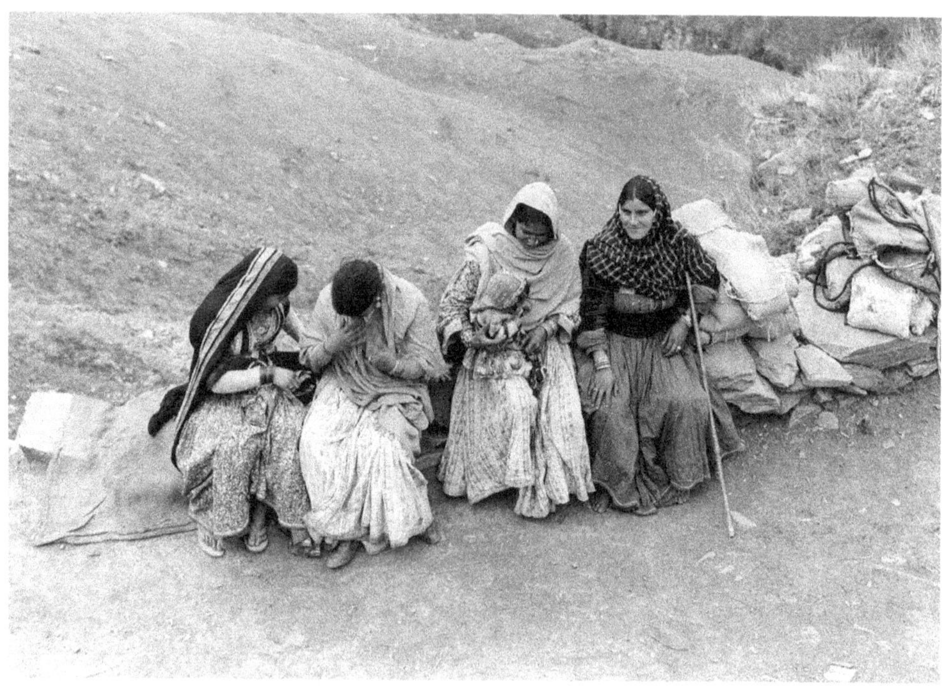

FIGURE 4.3. Four women in *luanchiri* made with hand-printed Rajasthani cloth, chatting and resting on a stone bench on their way down from Jalsu Pass toward Ravi Valley. They are on the spring (June) migration north from Kangra to Chamba. Photograph by Christina Noble, 1982, part of the collection held by Noble and the British Museum.

and heavy gold *nath* (nose ring) pinned in their noses. As I crossed the threshold into the singing room, the girls sprang up in shock. I was enveloped into the singing, clutched hands with sweaty palms. I clung onto them and was pulled down to the ground. I searched the room for Ira.

I found her sitting in the center of the room. She rushed over to greet me and pulled me from the melee into the clearer light of day. Ira looked so different from how I remembered her. Her thin wrists had thickened. Her cheeks were fuller, her nose adorned with a delicate nose ring wound with peacock metalwork. Her lips were painted a deep red. I noticed the swell of her belly straining against the gold paisley designs on her bright red suit. Her *mangal sutra* (marital necklace) hung from her neck.

Ira was tender with me. She held my upper arm and steered me to a quiet corner, where she clutched me to her. Ira explained that her own wedding had been only a few months earlier. Her husband was not the fiancé she had been chatting with on Facebook but someone else, a kind man who was gentle with her. He and his father do "driving work"—she pointed out the Suzuki Swift taxi up on the road. I told her I was sad that I hadn't come to her wedding.

"It's good you didn't come," she said. "I had such dark circles under my eyes. I had so much *tension* just before the wedding. I was the only one earning for the family at that time, and then I felt so guilty that I was about to leave."

It had taken her three years to save the money for her dowry and for the wedding, working in a café across the river.

"It wasn't a wedding like this one," she said, gesturing to the elaborate *mandap* (altar) set with awnings and a great throne for the bride and groom. "It was just normal, simple."

We gazed across the fields to where the bride was having her photo taken by a team of photographers. She posed with her *dupatta* (scarf) pulled low over her eyes in the field of wheat.

"But now I'm married in my own house, I'm OK, everything is OK. I know I need to take rest now, just be in my house and enjoy it."

We made our way down the road from the wedding, back to Uncle Keshav's house. We sat in the courtyard as the sun dipped, lighting up her gold-and-red *dupatta* from the back and shining through the delicate openings in her nose ring.

"When I got married, my father started taking some responsibility," Ira went on. "He stopped drinking, and he started working a bit, earning a bit. But this only happened after Shivani ran away."

Ira told me that, after the *ilaaj*, Shivani's health hadn't improved. She became more erratic and started sneaking off in the night. Their parents had reacted badly and jumped to arrange a marriage to a Hali boy from a few villages away. As much as Shivani protested, they would not change their minds. One morning Ira woke up, and Shivani was gone. Over time, they learned that she had run away with a Muslim boy from Dharamsala. Ira didn't know how they had met. All she knew was that now they lived in his family's house in the city, and Shivani had just given birth to a baby boy. Ira got out her phone to show me a picture of a small child wrapped up in a woolen sweater, cradled in the arms of a mother.

After Shivani left, however, her original fiancé's family was angry. They demanded that their son marry another of Shivani's sisters. Her own parents were wracked with shame and promised their youngest daughter, Aanchal, even though she was only seventeen. Aanchal had to go to the *panchayat* in the company of her parents to attest that she consented to marriage, even though she was under marriageable age. But she was excited, wanting the glamour and the intimacy and the clothes and the jewelry.

"I told Aanchal not to get married," Ira said as we sat in the courtyard, "but she did it for the *izzat* of my mother and father. She didn't listen to me. I said, 'You should get married later.' See, I'm twenty-seven years old. I have experienced lots of different things, and my mind has changed a lot. Aanchal is nine years younger than me; she is a very different age and personality. If you wait, you learn a lot of things—how to hold yourself, how to keep a house. But she just got married anyway."

Aanchal's marriage had not even lasted a year. Her husband beat her. Her husband's family beat her. She came home to her parents and eventually filed for divorce. Now Aanchal was also just "sitting at home," stuck between a present that was looping and slow and a future that seemed foggier and more fraught than ever.

5

Pagal

WHAT HAPPENS WHEN DISTRESS BECOMES DEVIANT?

Kapala

I first met Shruthi at a *nuala*—the sacred Shaivite devotional ritual where a goat is sacrificed to the Lord Shiva. I noticed Shruthi because she was standing on the edge of the circle of dancing women. She wore an unadorned black kurta and a thick black shawl, wrapped tightly around her shoulders. Where the other women moved synchronously as they sang the tale of Lord Shiva's marriage, Shruthi hovered at the threshold, moving with the group, then stepping out. Her eyes were elsewhere; she kept stopping to check her mobile phone. Like Shruthi, I was standing on the edge of the circle. She approached me as the music broke. She began to speak quickly, erratically. She gripped my arm, spilled my tea.

"When I was a child," she said, "they had a *nuala* especially for me." She looked me in the eye, considering for a moment. "When I was born, a priest

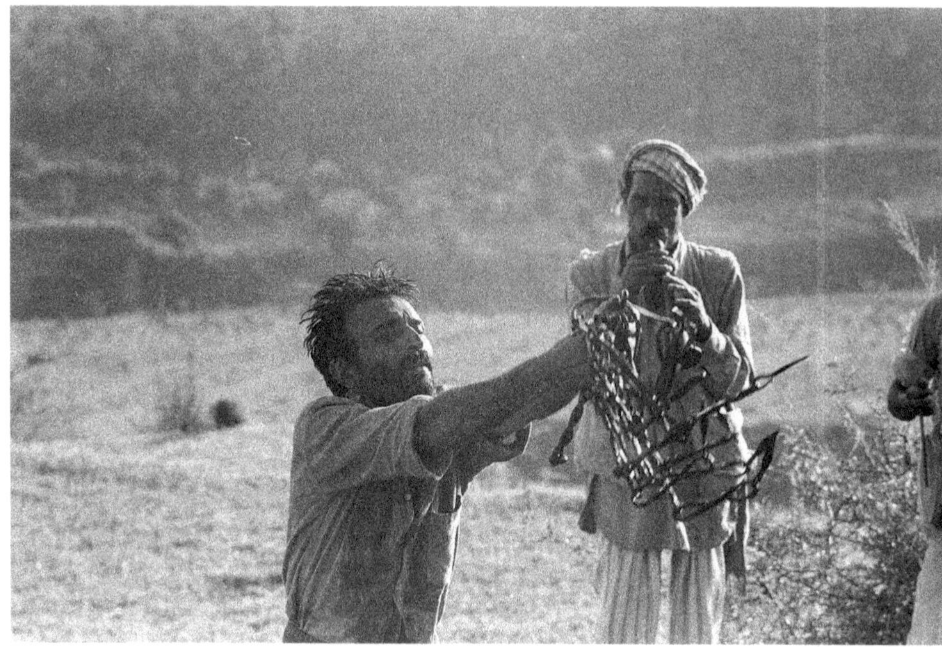

FIGURE 5.1. A man chosen by the village to serve as a vehicle for deities, known as a *gur*, is in a trance during a Jagra ritual. He whips himself with a *sangal* (metal whip). Photograph by Peter Phillimore, 1980.

came to my house. He told me that I wasn't allowed to brush or cut my hair for five years. He said that on my fifth birthday, I could cut my hair, and they could have a *nuala* for me." Her voice pitched. She began to rock as she spoke. "But on the fifth year, someone in my family died, so we couldn't have the *nuala* for another two years. I had dreadlocks then," she pointed to her smooth hair, imploring me to touch it. "I looked like a sadhu [ascetic]." She was close; I smelled her breath. When she bared her teeth, I noticed that the left incisor was decaying. She went on, looping and stuttering. When the music started again, she dipped into the dancing midway through her sentence. Cackling, she pulled me with her. Then again, abruptly, she stopped, sinking to the ground. She looked small, birdlike. Her hair had slipped from its clasp. Coquettishly, she pulled her shawl over her eyes like a new bride and batted her lashes. She seemed to appeal to the gaze of someone out of sight.

"You've met Shruthi," my friend Smriti whispered to me as I backed out of the circle. Smriti told me that Shruthi lived in a village close by and was married to Pankaj, a Gaddi Hali who worked at the hotel construction site near the slate mines. I came to know Shruthi very well. We had many fraught encounters. She would seek solace in me. I would cover for her. She would put my own reputation in the village at risk; I would put hers at risk. That night, however, Shruthi left me with only a cryptic remark.

"*Kapala*," she uttered when the dancing paused again. "I am a *kapala*. I look happy, beautiful, on the outside, but inside I have nothing. My husband has taken my heart. But now I earn the money for my children. My family gives me nothing." Later I asked Smriti what she meant. "*Kapala* means 'skull, or empty vessel,'" Smriti told me. *Kapali*, I learned, is another name for the divine and terrifying Lord Shiva, who is often pictured wearing a garland of skulls. It is also a name given to the ascetics, or sadhus, who devote their lives to him, wandering graveyards and cremation sites with a skull for an alms bowl.

From *Tension* to *Pagalpan*

Many Gaddi people told me that if one didn't manage their *tension*, then they could become *pagal*. *Pagal* is a Hindi term and was used by Gaddi people to describe a state of psychological and humoral imbalance that manifests in transgressive or erratic social behavior. *Pagal* (adjective) or *pagalpan* (noun) cannot be directly equated to the English terms *mad* or *madness*. Instead, like *tension* or other flexible terms like *stress* or *trauma*, it is a more fluid, contextual discourse that denotes an array of deviant behavioral, bodily, and mental states on the part of women, men, and children. In common parlance, the term was used humorously to indicate and even admire behavior that flirted at the edges of social acceptability or marked a change in norms—a mother laughing that her adolescent son was *pagal* for liking particular girls; a community health worker remarking that the younger generation of girls were *pagal* because they all demanded sanitary products or played sports. However, it was also applied to forms of mental distress that exceeded the normal conditions of life.

Distinctions in the meaning of *pagalpan* as distress loosely follow the division that I charted in chapter 1: between illnesses that are *sariri*, or natural bodily disruptions beyond human control, and afflictions caused by *opara* (black magic), *jadu* (witchcraft), or other forms of physical or emotional abuse caused by kin or affines. The *sariri* form of *pagal* was attributed to neurological imbalance, degeneracy, or brain injury. Such *pagal* people were also called *mental* or said to be afflicted by *dimagi ki problem* (problems of the mind). These terms were used to indicate problems caused by developmental delays, trauma to the head, dementia, epilepsy (*mirgi*), strokes (*attack*), or substance abuse. This kind of *pagal* was not necessarily gendered, nor was it related to a breakdown in kin or conjugal relationships, though it was said to cause their undoing. Importantly, this form of madness was somatically located in the brain and was not caused by imbalanced humors in the body. It could be treated through psychotropic medication sought at the psychiatric Outpatient Department at the Zonal Hospital or at psychiatric hospitals in urban centers. Rural families were unlikely to abandon kin who were afflicted by such conditions, despite the stigma that surrounded them. The assumption that someone's *pagal* was *sariri* worked to neutralize any moral transgression associated with their behavior, thus rendering it less dangerous.

A second form of *pagal*, caused by supernatural or human intervention, was more morally charged. It was used to signify the temporary divine madness of a holy person or person possessed by the divine, to signify socially deviant behavior, and to acknowledge the effects of neglect, trauma, or abuse that a person had experienced. "That man became *pagal* because his wife refused to feed him." "That woman is *pagal* because her husband beat her." In the most extreme cases, it was used as an accusation against those who engaged in morally, and particularly sexually, transgressive behaviors. No form of biomedical care—psychotropic medication or psychiatric consultation—was seen as effective or even applicable to this form of *pagalpan*, even if families first sought out psychiatric treatment. In all instances, a *pagal* person—whether temporarily or permanently mad—was in need of treatment or intervention from ritual healers or biomedical professionals, or a combination of the two. As Asaf Sharabi has argued in a similar Himalayan context, the politics of madness—or speculation as to whether a deviant person or people are authentically possessed by the divine, experiencing a psychopathology, or *pagal*—is a means by which socially subversive behavior is reflected on and neutralized.[1] Remarks about *pagal* people were not made publicly but were more often whispered along the rhythms of gossip, such that the assignation of blame or causality was speculative and slippery.

Rumors about *pagalpan* were deeply gendered. When applied to men, *pagal* indicated a state of mental or behavioral disorder that was often caused by a neglectful or sexually transgressive wife, sister, or mother. When applied to women, *pagalpan* indicated a state of disorder that was the result of tempestuousness, psychological weakness, and inadequate control over the balance in the household, the sexual body, and the mental state. In short, both the madness of men and the madness of women were the result of women's deviance.

THIS CHAPTER IS CONCERNED with unpicking the gendered relationalities of madness away from the determining frameworks of psychiatry or the law. Often, in ethnographic studies of madness or severe mental illness, we meet the afflicted figure *after* they have already been abandoned and cast out by their community. We meet them in institutional settings—the asylum, the hospital, the prison—or in medical records or legal case studies. The ethnographer's task is to piece together a disjointed narrative, as told by the afflicted figure themselves and their family, or by sifting through archival documents. Such approaches are revealing of the psychiatric discourses, legal categories, and bureaucratic processes that imprint or, in the Latourian formulation, "stabilize" the experience of madness.[2] However, when afflicted people are met in such settings, their biographies are written over by medical case files and legal proceedings such that people *become* their madness. To fetishize the experience of madness in this way, as anthropologist Tanya Luhrmann observes, does a terrible disservice to its pain by reducing it to its epistemological explanatory power.[3] To understand *pagalpan* in the context of the Gaddi relational theory of *tension*, it is necessary to overcome the "epistemic injustice," as Neil Armstrong puts it, drawing on philosopher Miranda Fricker, that devalues sufferers' own accounts of their distress.[4]

In this chapter I am less interested in the ways in which people already diagnosed with severe psychiatric conditions are further marginalized by psychiatric treatment encounters or state processes of what João Biehl has called *social abandonment*.[5] Instead, I focus on the social processes of stigmatization that generate the accusation of *pagalpan*, and the way in which such stigma is experienced by those who are considered *pagal*. In the words of the philosopher Ian Hacking, it is imperative to study madness through moral discourses of deviant and normal behavior as they are situated in what people do, how they live, and what larger material worlds they inhabit.[6] This requires a spatial point of departure that is not the psychiatric clinic or the ritual healing shrine but the intimate spaces of the household and neighborhood from where suspicions of madness grow and impress on particular subjectivities. It requires a temporal point of departure that is not retrospective (looking backward on the life of a subject from a present that is determined by a diagnosis of madness) but dynamic (looking through the incremental relational shifts through which a person's behavior is stigmatized).

To gain this wider lens, I draw on an alternative, largely forgotten, anthropological conversation on "deviance." Both psychiatry and the anthropology of mental health have an uneasy relationship with the concept of deviance. Deviance is most often associated with gendered and sexual positionalities that depart from the normative. The elision of sexual deviance with psychiatric aberration in diagnoses like hysteria has its roots in nineteenth-century psychiatry's attempts to explain away superstitious or magical etiologies of sexual transgression in favor of modern scientific accounts. These elisions were codified when the first *Diagnostic and Statistical Manual* (DSM) was published in 1952. The category of sexual deviation specifically included transvestism, homosexuality, pedophilia, fetishism, and sexual sadism.[7] Today, as we look back on such understandings of sexuality and gender through a mature anthropology of sexuality, armed with the tools of queer theory, deviance seems unsexy—antiquated at best and stigmatizing at worst. However, as queer studies scholars Gayle Rubin and Heather Love point out, our contemporary understandings of sex and gender, stigma, and resistance are greatly indebted to "deviance studies." As Love reminds us, midcentury American "urban reformers and academic sociologists [were] concerned with patterns of settlement and symptoms of social disorder."[8] Sociologists like Erving Goffman, John Gagnon, Howard Becker, and Esther Newton conducted in-depth empirical studies of "permanently stigmatized groups" from marginal spaces like cruising spots, gay bars, and tea rooms in "more or less diseased or deviant zones" of US cities.[9] In their studies, Love tells us, the outsider figure is fetishized by the bird's-eye view that the researcher takes—refusing to identify with the subject of study. However, Love argues that there is something to be said for the way they treat the views of "deviants" as of equal importance as those of "respectable citizens" and "authorities," and for the way in which they disrupted the medical and psychological framings of sexual deviance by situating such positionalities in relational processes of stigmatization, labeling, and discrimination. Deviance studies were rightly critiqued in the 1970s by Black and Marxist scholars who began to break down sociology's epistemic frameworks by aligning with the "underdogs" and with the wider turn to language and social constructionism. However, both Love and Rubin trace how the contemporary anthropology of sexuality is formed on the back of these earlier studies, arguing that the amnesia toward these genealogical roots renders queer theory blind to its own power dynamics.

In this chapter I follow Rubin and Love in finding something productive in the attention to incremental, relational dynamics of social exclusion and stigma that earlier studies of deviance pioneered. Seeing *pagalpan* as a form of deviance rather than mental illness has an empirical accuracy that allows me to attend to the ways in which extreme distress is generated through forms of relational rupture or breakdown, rather than determined by psychiatric diagnostics in this case. Through the lens of deviance, and a particular attention to stigma, I argue that *pagalpan* is best understood as a social process of exclusion based on gendered, casted, and classed positionality, rather than a psychological condition based on psychic symptoms or their psychiatric classification. In previous chapters the expression of *tension*, *kamzori* (weakness), or other conditions both registers the pressure of such relational injury and allows women to push back against and renegotiate their relationships such that they are able to cling to fantasies of domesticity, intimacy, belonging, or generational flourishing. In this chapter we explore what happens when such relationships break down as a result of conflict, violence, or abuse.

In these instances, people, and particularly women in unhappy marriages, become the focus of intense suspicion and speculation on the part of neighbors and kin. Under the pressure of this gaze, a woman's behavior might become, or come to be seen as, deviant. It is in these moments that they are vulnerable to whispers that they are *pagal*. As we will see, these whispers are not totalizing acts of discrimination or dehumanization. Instead, they work on one hand to acknowledge the trauma that a woman has been through, to mark her unmet needs or desires and the ways she has been wronged by her husband or affines. On the other, such whispers work to further stigmatize her behavior and to render her more marginal. These instances, as Sarah Pinto puts it in her ethnography of women's madness in Agra, dramatize the axes of life that are very normal, if in heightened form.[10] Herein, women become caught in webs of relations that produce no coherent position in kinship.[11] The fantasies of domesticity, intimacy, and belonging that structure such kinship relations become simulated or overdetermined, or simply no longer hold. As such, the deviant behavior of *pagal* women works to open a gap in the aesthetics of patriarchal life, a fissure from which possibilities for living otherwise might emerge. We find *pagal* subjectivities far from abject but instead replete with dangerous potencies that exceed dominant patriarchal ideologies. Let us return to Shruthi to watch how such processes of stigmatization play out.

The Toilet

I was inspecting the foul trail of plastic wrappers that littered a *nali* (drain, stream) that cut through the village of Thera when I heard someone shriek my name. Shankar and I had climbed down to the lower outcrops of the lower-caste hamlet with our two dogs. I didn't realize that this was where Shruthi lived until she came running out from her courtyard with the same ratty black shawl streaming out behind her. Shruthi's mud house backed directly onto the drain, such that the stench wafted into her home on the southerly breeze. I could smell it as I turned my head up to see her leaning over the gate to clasp my hand, pulling me inside.

"I hoped you would pass by and come into my house," she panted. This time her words were not cryptic. She was direct, pragmatic in her tone. "I wanted to ask if you needed someone to come and clean for you, someone to do your housework. I could start right away. I need the money, you see; my husband is useless, and I have four children to provide for, all on my own." She fiddled nervously with her hair, then with the clasp on her wallet. She didn't wait for me to answer before she turned her attention to Shankar.

"Look at this space." She pointed to a shallow patch of overturned dirt next to the courtyard gate. She grabbed a spade that was stuck into the dirt and began to drive it violently into the soil. "I want to build a septic tank and a toilet for my daughters; they have to go and use the *nali*, even at night, to shit or piss." She pummeled the spade into the broken earth at random. "The men might come to watch them." She winced, gesturing to the tea shop at the base of the hamlet that that was well known for serving home-brewed desi alcohol to slate miners and construction workers on their way back to the village. "I have to do it myself; my husband or my mother-in-law won't help me." She began to fire off a litany of questions to Shankar: How much is the cost of labor? How much would it cost to get some local men in to help her build it? Would he come and help? Did he know anyone who would do it for her? She only had a budget of ten thousand rupees. Shankar didn't have the chance to get a word in before she launched on.

"My father-in-law gave me some money before he died, but I have to use it for everything; they give me nothing, they do nothing for me." She gasped for air. "For seventeen years I have faced this without respite." We heard a lashing of expletives coming from the other side of the courtyard. Shruthi's mother-in-law came lumbering out of her kitchen, dragging her bad leg behind her. She shooed us away, screaming about how our dogs would piss on her flowerbeds. We scurried up the hill, the dogs following. I never saw that toilet built.

SHRUTHI WAS FROM CHAMBA, the Himachali district on the other side of the majestic Dhaula Dhar range, more remote than Kangra, but a sacred land for the Gaddis. She was also from a different caste to that of her husband. Shruthi was an upper-caste Rajput, from a reputable flock-owning family. She was the eldest of five children, two sisters and three brothers. She was in ninth standard, and fifteen years old, when she met Pankaj, whose Hali family was living for a time in the region. They fell in love, and despite her family's wishes, they eloped. Pankaj's family returned to their home in Kangra, and Shruthi went with them. Her own family cut contact. By her sixteenth birthday, she was pregnant with her elder daughter, Beena, and was living in Kangra with her in-laws. When she first arrived in her *sasural*, her husband's village, she had been hopeful. She was deeply in love, and her husband was adoring. But this romance soon evaporated.

"Shruthi was so different when she came, before it all started," Sita, Shruthi's neighbor, remarked one afternoon, as we were drinking tea together. Sita had promised to show me some photos of old days in the village. We chatted as she spread out the photos on the crisp sheet. I began to slowly rifle through them. A picture of Sita's husband the day he left for work in Delhi. Of her sister in traditional Gaddi dress dancing at a function in Dharamsala. Then a picture of a woman looking directly into the camera. She stood against a metal mesh, like the fencing that lines a prison or zoo enclosure. She was dressed in a purple suit and a cheap red *dupatta* (scarf). This was Shruthi on her wedding day. Her hands were adorned to the elbow with bangles, nails painted red. She held them aloft, as if not quite sure where to put them. She clutched a tissue. The *sindoor* (vermilion) in the part of her hair looked thick and fresh.

Adjust Karna Parega

As explored in chapter 3, the movement from exchange marriage to prestige marriage that has occurred over the past fifty years, from large households to nuclear households, and toward legalized Hindu marriage, has located intimacy in the permanent conjugal bond. As Kriti Kapila shows, since the late twentieth century, the breakdown of marriage—in elopement, divorce, second marriage, extramarital sex—is no longer tolerated as it was in previous generations.[12] The unyoking of caste distinctions from economic divisions within the pastoral economy, and the adoption of Hindu Nationalist principles, has made marriage a key arbiter of caste superiority, rendering intercaste and interfaith marriage deeply disgraceful. Marital relations become, in Nate Roberts's words, "moral faultlines" that, like geological fault lines, articulate the contradictions, instabilities, or anxieties in moral worlds in ways that are hidden from view.[13] Those who flaunt caste or class restrictions are the source of much speculation and stigma.

Gaddi people speak of the need to make a marriage work through the idiom of "adjustment."[14] "You have to adjust [to marriage]; it takes time," Minoti, a Hali neighbor, explained to me as we sat on her porch one evening.

> The thinking in this family is different from the thinking in that family. You have to restrain yourself until you understand the setup in that family; your thinking isn't free. This is married life; this life is different

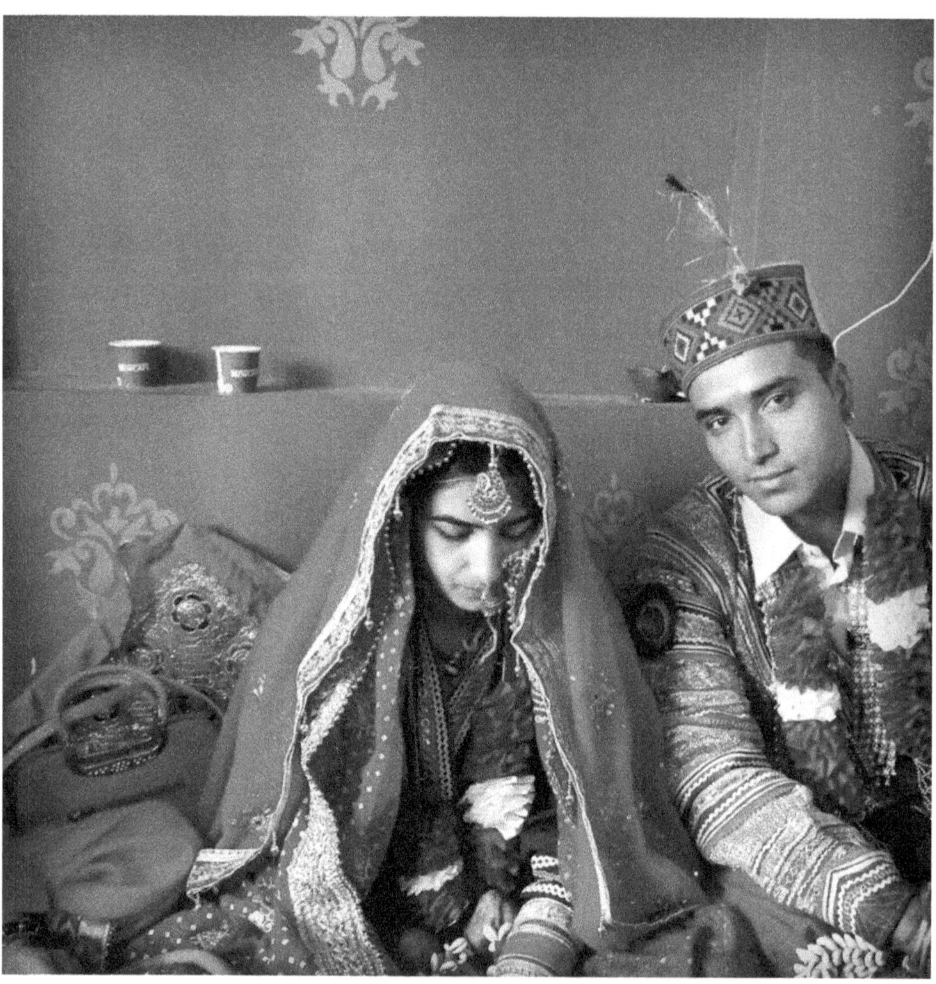

FIGURE 5.2. A new bride after her wedding day, in her husband's house. Photograph by Nikita Kaur Simpson, 2018.

> from the life before marriage. But married life can be beautiful too. Before marriage, everything is open; it is your own, at your own choice you can eat what you like, wear what you like, get up, sit, and sleep as you like. Before marriage, if I felt like sleeping anytime, I would go to sleep, but after marriage, you can't. Everything is going on in the house; people are fighting in the house. Before marriage, I didn't cook anything. . . . After marriage, I get tired but can't sleep. Life is very different.

For women, the path of marriage is emotionally fraught, as they must grapple with their own in-betweenness while habituating to their marital home.[15]

After marriage, a woman is expected to subjugate her own desires and needs to those of her marital family. She must wear the signs of her constricted sexuality—marital jewelry, tied hair, vermilion applied to her parting (*sindoor*), and a veil in front of her male affines (*ghoonghat*).[16] The process of adjusting to a new home is fraught; one is under the intense gaze of immediate and extended family members who might find fault in every move.

A newly married woman is also expected to become pregnant within the immediate period following her marriage, preferably with a boy child. Only when a woman has had boy children is she integrated into her marital family, cementing her status in her new household. If her first child is a girl, her family is often disappointed. If her second child is a girl, she might be shamed. Kiran, an *anganwadi* (government daycare) worker, explained the traumas of these first years to me: "If they have one girl and she is pregnant, then they worry about the second baby. If that baby is also a girl . . . *Bechari* [poor thing]. . . . She worries, What will my mother- and father-in-law say if it is a girl, how will we look after a girl? She has all of these worries during the birth of her baby. But this shouldn't happen; if the lady takes *tension*, then the baby will be affected. Whatever is in the mother's mind will also be in the baby's mind."

Abortion is common, particularly in the upper castes—clinics in Pathankot are accessed illegally and secretly by many Gaddi families who can afford it, or it is forced through nonclinical means. Kiran went on:

> But there is another thing in this village, not just in this village, in all places. If you have two girls, [the pregnant women] will only come after three months [of pregnancy]. We don't come to know when [they get abortions] done, but they will register when they are pregnant and find out. If it is a girl, then they will get the abortion done. They will say that it just miscarried by itself. You can't tell whether they have done it themselves or not. How can it miscarry itself? But we don't have any proof. They do get depressed. The people in the house make them do these things. Then she gets depressed. How can the mother recover if the whole family is after her? It's wrong to do it. Then they will get pain around the uterus and infection there. They become very weak [*kamzor*] inside. If this happens again and again, they get very weak and depressed. If they get weak inside, then what can we do for them? If they get it done repeatedly and they get pregnant again, then they miscarry because they aren't strong enough to carry the child. This is the main problem. Then they can't have children. It's not her life; it's her family who does this.

> They put a lot of pressure on her. Their thinking isn't good; that's why they have problems. Some people have good thinking; they have two girls, and they say, That's OK. But some people's thinking isn't good; they have two girls, three girls, four girls because they need a boy. What can you do?

This process of adjustment is particularly difficult for women who have no social support from their *maike*, or natal home. Such women experience an extreme social isolation, for they don't have the protection of their fathers or brothers. It is also made difficult if their *sasural*, or affines, oppose or resent the marriage. They are considered more inauspicious, their bodily substances incompatible with this new place. For such women, like Shruthi, the trials of marriage seem to multiply.[17]

TWO PREGNANCIES FOLLOWED SHRUTHI'S first—another girl, Pinky, before she finally had a son, Rohit. It was during this time that the beatings started. Everyone in the village knew that Shruthi had suffered immense horrors at the hands of her husband and mother-in-law. Shruthi was one of the few women who spoke directly about the difficulties that she had experienced during her marriage, and about the violence she had suffered. "My mother-in-law is a horrible woman," she muttered. "Bahut ganda kaam [Very dirty work]." Shruthi spoke plainly of how she was beaten and locked in the house, how she would watch her children play from the window.

Shruthi left her husband when her father-in-law died. When I met her, she had been separated from him for three years. She was living in the same compound as her mother-in-law and husband, in a set of dank mud rooms across the courtyard from their concrete house. Shruthi's three daughters lived with her. They weren't allowed to use the toilet in the main house, so resorted to the stinking drain that ran along the side of the village. Her son stayed with his father and was fed and cared for by his grandmother. Pankaj was still a drunk and didn't earn much from the odd jobs he did—serving as a security guard for a local hotel, working on construction sites. Shruthi earned her own money—cooking at a campsite, cleaning rooms in a hotel across the river, doing laundry at a hostel higher up in the valley. She complained that her husband came to each of her workplaces drunk, pining for her, hitting her, blubbering to her employers. One employer told me that they had to fire her to stop him from making a scene again. Shruthi had been to the *panchayat* and local feminist nongovernmental organizations (NGOs) for legal advice. They sent her to the *nari adalat*, women's court, but her case was thrown out for lack of consistent evidence of battery.[18]

AS IN SHRUTHI'S CASE, the initial romantic attachment following a marriage sometimes collapses under the weight of strained relations with affines, financial insecurity, infertility, miscarriages, forced abortions, and the absence of a boy child. Women's hopes of intimacy, respect, and mutual care are shattered by husbands whose frustrations boil over. As we see with Shruthi, the obligation to adjust persists through the experience of domestic violence.

Once, during a visit to the village beauty parlor, I struck up a conversation with a woman getting her eyebrows threaded. She was a Gaddi Rajput woman, Sukriti, with two grown-up children. Her husband worked in the water department in Dharamsala. I also knew her sister, Nandini, who lived in a beautiful concrete house in the village below the one where I lived. Nandini was known for both her beauty and the violence that she had suffered at the hands of her husband and her mother-in-law. When I passed by her house, she was often crouching in the small waterfall washing clothes. She would come running to the road to whisper to me of her *tension*. In the parlor that day, I tentatively began to ask Sukriti some questions about marriage and motherhood. Interested, the other ladies in the parlor joined in the conversation. I pitched to them a number of scenarios: A woman whose husband was an alcoholic, unable to provide for his children. A woman abused from the outset of marriage by her mother-in-law. A woman whose kind and loving husband had become violent after the birth of their first girl child. In all situations, the women were adamant that the woman must stay with her husband. They screwed up their faces and shook their heads—of course she must stay; she must adjust (*adjust karna parega*). They were unsympathetic, agreeing with each other that they should get on with things.

As the psychiatrist Edith Gahleitner has also found in Kangra, instances of domestic abuse often surround domestic acts.[19] Husbands and affines abused women for giving them bad food or not keeping the house clean. Beatings were symptomatic of the failure to be a "good wife." Indeed, the imprint of this violence is present in the collective fantasy of domesticity. In drama workshops I conducted with adolescent girls from the village, participants were given prompts and asked to act out a classic scenario in their home. The participants acted out a familiar scene—a man drinking with his friends, returning to his house, and demanding food from his wife for himself and the other men, his wife dutifully providing. Her husband, unhappy with the food, throws it across the room and pulls his wife by the hair, screaming abuse. Gahleitner also found that women left their husbands only if there was a threat to their life or to the lives of their children, after which point the woman's depression was likely to peak. Living in their natal home or alone, they faced the shame and stigma of a failed marriage and of being an unwanted burden on their natal kin.

Recent progressive legislative shifts, while providing recourse to statutory support for some, only worked to further stigmatize others. Most specifically, the Domestic Violence Act (2005) and the outcomes of the Verma Commission Report empowered women and their families financially and legally to leave abusive relationships.[20] However, such legislation is also used to contest the legitimacy of marriages that are deemed aberrant—elopements become kidnappings, intercaste marriages are annulled on grounds of abuse or dowry torture—undermining women's choices.[21] Appeal to such legislation in the village is seen as an act of individualistic cunning, and the veracity of women's claims is often disputed. As one policewoman explained:

> Their husband beats them; maybe there is less dowry, so they beat them. Or about money, the husbands don't give money to the wives for household and the children's education. If [this] is reported, then [the courts] make [the husband] give a certain amount of money to his wife . . . every month. This is very common, but some people just tell lies. . . . When a lady is raped, then they get four lakhs from the state. So, you know what ladies do? They tell a lie about it. Many say this, that they were with someone, and they were fighting, like if a boy and girl are living together, and then the boy's off with someone else, then if he is not fulfilling her demands, and she might say that he has done this with me. But this is wrong because they were living together because they wanted to live together. The court is always in the lady's favor. They know they will get this money.

Within this context, a woman who is suspected of sexual exploits and who has refused to fall back into line when she is called out is dangerous in a new way. She who is actively resistant to the reprimands or violence that is inflicted on her, who is unable to be reintegrated into the marital household—whose *izzat* (honor, respectability) cannot be domesticated—is seen as a threat.

New Anxieties

Smriti and I were passing through Shruthi's hamlet when a flash of cobalt blue caught my eye. Shruthi was standing on the threshold of her kitchen, holding up a brilliant blue kurta top. "Hey!" She called us over. She danced with the kurta, twirling it around and cocking her head. "Do you like it?" she sang and beckoned us over. "I have a new job, at a school in the next valley. This is my uniform!" We climbed the stairs to her kitchen. The floors were well swept, but the shelves were bare; unlike in other kitchens, there were no packets of lentils or coconut biscuits. Shruthi handed Pinky a ten-rupee note from her wallet and rushed her to pick up a packet of tea leaves and biscuits to serve us. Her hands shook as she set the pot on to boil for the tea, and when Pinky arrived back, she added only one teaspoonful of leaves. She didn't look at us as she spoke:

> It's very difficult for me, very difficult. Here, nobody gives me anything; nobody speaks to me. These days, I can't go anywhere in the village without people saying something about me. Who have you been going with? they ask. I just even go to [the market] to get some vegetables, and they say, Where has she been? Who has she been with? My husband gets so angry, so angry, he says, Don't go now. . . . Because I don't have a *maike* here, I have nowhere to go. . . . The people in this village are so dirty.

"How is your work?" I asked her.

"Yes, it is good work," she replied, taking care to put the silver teacups on a tray before she passed them to us. "But I get very little money, and the expenses [of the household] are a lot. . . . Everyone needs something; I have to get everything for the children, every morning [there is something more]." Shruthi began to speak about how this condition of constant rumor and gossip made her ill.

"I have fear. I have fear inside me; I don't know what's happened. All the time. . . . I feel better [if I speak about my problems], but people listen to my problems, and they don't understand. The voice comes into their ears, but they don't understand." Smriti asked if she ever thought of leaving her husband properly, getting a divorce and leaving the village. This time she looked up, straight at us, defiantly.

"I must do it. I have to go and get it done in the court, but it costs a lot, ten thousand rupees. I will get expenses if the divorce goes through from the court." Shruthi was worried, though, about where she would go if the divorce went through.

> If I go back [to Chamba] to find work, then all of those people will ask what has happened. What's happened to her? If I go back there and take quarters in their house, they will say—how many years have gone past? She is their oldest daughter; she is too old to stay here. What can she do? They will say very bad things about me. I have so much *izzat*, but they will say I have none. They won't keep me. Those people get upset if I am inside,

> or if I am outside. I think I will go and rent a house here. My children can choose themselves if they come with me or stay with their father.

The pain welled up. She began to whisper:

> When I was married, I tried to do the right thing. They gave me so many utensils to wash; I had so much to do. I was so scared of them. I cooked so much for so many people. . . . My hands were cracked. I was only sixteen. When I was seventeen, Beena was born. I washed so many clothes. They would all hit me, all hurt me. They would only leave me such a small amount of food in a bowl, and I would have to just eat that and sleep. They were so dirty. . . . Here in this village they only want this from women. Have children. Do the cow's work. If you do anything else, they talk about you.

New forms of mobility and employment also generated significant moral panic and invited intimate partner or kin violence, as they were seen to offer new opportunities for supposed impropriety. Women who had to work, and particularly those who worked in Dharamsala, Kangra, or McLeod Ganj, were considered suspect. McLeod—a tourist center and the residence of the Tibetan government in exile—was conceived as a place of debauchery where tourists and gangs from the plains engaged in sex work and drug dealing. Such accusations reached any woman who was spatially mobile. Women who breached the boundaries of the home and the village, particularly after dark, were the butt of much speculation. The intrusion of seasonal workers, tourists, and louts from the plains necessitated an extra level of vigilance for women and those who sought to "protect" them from others and from their own temptations. The intimate and surveilling gaze of men in the village served to both sexualize women and secure their *izzat*. When I conducted workshops with young women, however, asking them to draw maps of the village space around their house and shade in the areas where they felt safe or unsafe, it was not only the outsiders who caused them anxiety. These young women saw the tea shops that dotted the village, filled with local men from their own caste drinking home-brewed alcohol, as just as unsafe as the areas where men from other castes or from outside the village tended to dwell.

THE USE OF MOBILE phones and social media was also seen to facilitate aberrant behavior. A woman who was seen on the phone too often, or who took photos that were considered too provocative, was considered dangerous and

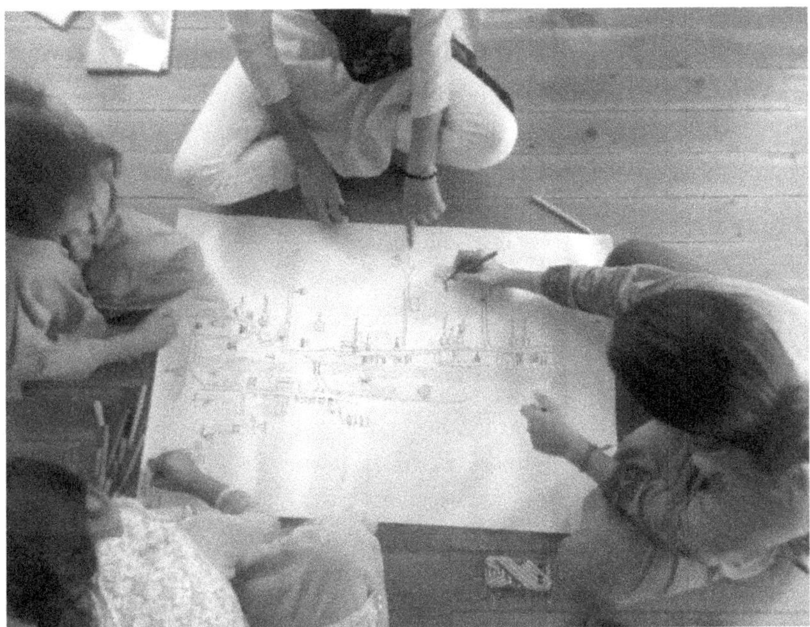

FIGURE 5.3. Girls draw a map of their village during a workshop. They have shaded the emotions they feel in different places in different colors. They note that they feel scared and unsafe close to the temple, where many men spend time drinking in tea shops and cat-calling is common. Photograph by Nikita Kaur Simpson, 2018.

suspected of sexual impropriety. Young women's phones were checked for secret boyfriends. Girls were told stories of visiting men from other caste and religious groups who would attempt to contact them via their mobile phones. Such "wrong number" relationships were a source of excitement and potential for women due to their combination of emotional intimacy and physical distance.[22] The mobile phone was seen as a euphemism for disallowed intimacies.[23] However, such a euphemism was not used to explain away these illicit affairs. Instead, a woman's use of a mobile phone was an excuse for a moral reprimand, as I saw in the case of my landlord's relationship with Shruthi.

"THAT WOMAN IS ALWAYS on her phone." My neighbor, Uncle Keshav, would often shake his head as he spoke of Shruthi. Indeed, Shruthi often came over to my house under the guise of dropping off a small gift or wanting a cup of tea. She would then make a lengthy and animated phone call from our kitchen. One day

I spotted her getting off the evening bus against the summer sunset. She shouted up from the road, asking if she might come in for tea. She was particularly raucous that day; she laughed gleefully, pinched my cheeks, and slapped her hands together. She kept pulling her peach-colored scarf around her face and then flinging it to the ground. Usually when I met her, I had company. Perhaps her intensity struck me so much that day because I was alone with her. I didn't have to ask her any questions; her news came pouring out of her.

"I don't have much to do with the children anymore. I have totally escaped the household. I don't have time for them, and I don't see what they do. I am always at work at my new job." Shruthi had been fired from the job at the school when her husband came to the premises drunk. She was now working as a cleaner at a pool hall in the Tibetan compound that borders the village. The hall was busy these days, with Tibetan young men who came to drink beer.

"They all come to see me!" She giggled. "They come to speak with me, especially Bhai [a local businessman]." Shruthi recounted how Bhai had visited her last week and remarked on how beautiful she was. Shruthi laughed uncontrollably and slapped my hand again. "But my family aren't happy. They say—you are always roaming about, getting back late, always on the phone." She stopped and looked at me, grinning. "Where is Hugo? I haven't seen him on the bus." Shruthi and my partner, Hugo, had sometimes met on the bus into Dharamsala when she was on her way to her job in the school. I explained that Hugo had bought a motorbike and now didn't need to catch the daily bus into town.

"People are always asking, Where is your boyfriend?!" She dissolved into a fit of laughter. She noticed that I was getting uncomfortable. She grabbed my wrist. "I am OK now, you know," she said. "My *tension* is OK. There is nothing wrong with me. But Pankaj is *ganda* [dirty]; his mind is so bad. We are always fighting. If I hadn't run away, I would have been literate. One person I'll never forgive in my life is this man." This was the last time that Shruthi came to visit me. My landlord soon realized how she was using my house to make phone calls and forbade her from visiting. He wouldn't want to be suspected of facilitating this kind of behavior.

Between Pity and Blame

People in the hamlet pitied Shruthi. Her troubles, especially the frequent and public fights that she had with her mother-in-law, were well known to her neighbors. They tutted over the uselessness of her husband, who could often be found singing, drunk, through the village streets of a Saturday morning.

But this pity often tipped into more malicious remarks: "She got what she deserved"; "She should never have married him in the first place"; "She should have found a way of dealing with that witch, of adjusting to that house." These malicious remarks tipped into suspicions and rumors: "You know, it's because she was having an affair with her father-in-law"; "She's always running off to the city; who knows if she has someone there"; "She uses that house as if it's a brothel." As her behavior became more erratic, and more overtly sexualized, these rumors became accusations of *pagal*.

THE SUSPICION THAT A woman was *pagal* was most commonly leveled against women whose marriages had frayed. People were accused of crossing the threshold from *tension* to *pagal* if they were unable to sustain their relationships and meet the expectations of kin and affines. As an illocutionary act, the label worked to blame women for their failure to hold together broken kinship relations, to adjust, or to remain silent. But it also worked to acknowledge the trauma that they might have experienced at the hands of their husband or affinal family. Instances of reproductive failure, miscarriage, infertility, the loss of a child or forced sex-selective abortion, widowhood, separation, or divorce left women vulnerable to becoming *pagal*. Such women were vulnerable through both domestic and structural violence—harassment, discrimination, social isolation, stigma, economic vulnerability, feelings of worthlessness.[24] Such traumatic events might be seen as relational injuries rather than purely intrapsychic or structural ones, where worlds of kinship are unmade in pain.[25] Herein, *pagal* might be seen as a socially sanctioned and culturally inflected means of acknowledging such trauma and its impact on a woman's mind and body—articulating both pity for a woman who is failed by her kin *and* critique of a woman unable to adjust and meet the expectations placed on her.

SHRUTHI'S TRANSITION IN THE eyes of her neighbors from a subject of pity to an object of disdain occurred over seventeen years. At first, her neighbors told me that they worried about her. The fights in that house were frequent, theatrical, and public. She was seen as young and foolish to have eloped. But she was also seen as unlucky to have found her way into such a turbulent family, where Pankaj's mother was notoriously scathing—known for her quick tongue and agility with a stick. Some said that Pankaj's mother was a *dain* (witch), that she knew the spells of *opara*. Others said that she kept poison scattered on her fields for any dog who came sniffing. As Shruthi hardened under the violence, she began to fight back. The more public the fighting grew, the more isolated Shruthi became. The village women often called the police in the beginning, but when they arrived, Shruthi denied being beaten. She didn't want to lose her husband, they sighed. She still loved him.

As Shruthi's behavior became more erratic, they began to whisper about the affairs she was having. How else would she have so much money? How else could she afford to leave her husband? How else did she have the money for that smartphone, those earrings, those blue jeans? She was always on that phone, they muttered, like a choir in a Greek play. Her husband was admittedly useless. He didn't protect her from his mother, he couldn't choose; they pursed their lips. But this didn't excuse her for entertaining other men. They would come to her in the dead of night, the women conjectured. Wasn't she seen in the back of a car on the way to Dharamshala? Shruthi's daily journey to and from whichever place she was currently working at served as fodder for rumor. Indeed, she played the part well. She would dress up coquettishly, lining her lips a little too much. She would always return after dark.

Shruthi didn't behave like other Gaddi married women: She was effusive, flirtatious; she screamed in public; she let her children run free. Pankaj was also considered in some way *pagal*. He was often found singing old Gaddi songs in a drunken stupor up and down the village road. He was known for his unpaid debts, his unsolicited sexual advances toward the village women, and his inability to keep his wife in line. He was even rumored to have beaten up his own uncle over a minor disagreement. However, Pankaj himself was not blamed for his deviant and even violent behavior. Instead, Shruthi was chastised for her inability to adjust to her marital home, sending her husband to alcoholism as a result of her failure as a mother to his children, along with her extramarital sexual exploits. It was her supposedly selfish failure to care for her husband and children that led the village to label her as *pagal*.

The nexus of violence that engulfed this household led others to avoid it. As if her deviance were polluting or contagious, Shruthi's neighbors discouraged me from visiting her and from playing with her children. If I spent too much time with Shruthi, neighbors would talk, and I could even be cursed by some kind of *opara*. Shruthi's madness had some kind of dark power over the community that threatened to undo the careful work of *izzat*.

Contagious Madness

A close reading of Shruthi's case against others reveals that *pagal* is not only a stigmatizing discursive label or accusation. Instead, *pagal* works as a form of miasmic pollution, penetrating the flesh and substances of the deviant body in ways that are both symbolic and material. Like *tension*, it is an embodied and relational quality that seems to move between the body of an afflicted woman and those of her intimate partners, children, or kin. This is seen in the way that Shruthi's neighbors frame Pankaj's alcoholism as an affliction that has emanated from her body and come to afflict her husband's. It inspired a particular fear on the part of neighbors that warranted avoidance of Shruthi and her family. Bhrigupati Singh and Pratap Sharan frame this kind of relational, contagious distress as *asrat* (an "effect" in Hindi-Urdu; "difficulty" in Arabic). "Rather than being located solely in an individual body or brain," they contend, an *asrat* "affliction is conceived as transferrable across bodies, most often a household or a kinship group."[26] The core feature of an *asrat* illness is that it often begins with "a threat to existence arising from a disorder of intimate otherness, which may initially appear as a *shaq* (doubt/suspicion) or a kind of certainty in the perception of psychic and economic injuries and conflicts with intimates such as spouses, siblings, neighbors, kin, or business associates."[27] In the case of Shruthi's *pagalpan*, this existential threat is libidinal—the threat of the female sexuality, or *shakti*, usually channeled into conjugal and affinal relations, becomes unbounded by the confines of kinship. While it is absorbed by and emanates from the body of the woman herself, it is felt as a sense of distress and disorder by a woman's husband and affinal kin. We can see how this works in another case of *pagalpan*.

TANU WAS THE WIFE of the Dogri slate miner, Tinku. Over the past few years, Tinku had come to be known as a *sharabi* (alcoholic)—depressed and unable to work. He attributed his condition to his *pagal* wife. Tanu, Tinku told Shankar and me, had been *pagal* since before marriage. Someone had cursed her with *jadu*, and the curse had lived in her body and been brought into his household. When they got married, the *jadu* got much stronger and began to affect him.

"If you are single," he explained, "and you have *jadu*, [and] then you get married, it also gets married and becomes more powerful. It comes to feed on two people, on the whole *ghar* [household]." His family had done a lot of different rituals to try and protect themselves from such curses before he had married and afterward, when it became clear that Tinku's new bride was afflicted. These rituals were aimed at firming up the boundaries of the house and exorcising the *jadu* from her body. But Tinku's wife became pregnant soon after the wedding, and her condition worsened.

"When she was pregnant, she took a knife and tried to stab her baby. Maybe some *cela* [ritual healer] that we took her to took advantage of her. It was some *najaiz faida* [abuse]. Maybe she was *chalak* [sly] and had some [sexual] relation with someone." After Tinku's wife had the baby, she settled. But then Tinku began to become affected.

"Many problems began to happen," he recounted. "I didn't have work, and I didn't have anyone to share with. Her *pagalpan* affected me a lot, and the idea that she had been with someone else." Tinku began to get depressed and to drink. His wife became frustrated with him in a new way. She became afflicted by *ghar ki tension*—feelings of unidentifiable pain and fatigue settled in her body, and she received regular visits in her dreams from the Jungle Raja. They sent their son to Shimla to live with Tinku's sister because neither of them could look after him and he wasn't going to school. Before long, Tanu found a new man to be with. She ran away with him to Darjeeling, and Tinku had to travel there to get her back. Now, she had returned to the house and had settled again. She spent her days doing housework and looking after Tinku and his mother. Her son returned, and her madness abated. But the house was still afflicted by *ghar ki tension*, Tinku had again been hospitalized with a snakebite, and he admitted that he was still taking psychotropic medication for depression.

Midway through Tinku's story, his wife quietly entered the room. She had gone to a neighboring house to fetch milk and now sat with it cradled in her lap. Tinku looked up at her when she entered and went on with the story. She set down the milk and began to knit. Her body craned forward; she seemed to hover over me, as if she had something to add, something to tell. But she was stopped by a sharp look from her mother-in-law, who had also come to sit on the other side of Tinku. As we were leaving, Tanu followed me out of the house and down the steps toward the gate. She caught my arm. "Could you find me a job in an office?" she whispered.

Blueprints for Madness

The cases of Shruthi and Pankaj, and of Tanu and Tinku, reveal an important relational impasse that sits at the heart of Gaddi marriage. In both cases, women who become *pagal* are blamed for failing to adjust, to discipline their desires to those of their husband and affines. However, men and affines are also blamed for and become vulnerable to the unmet desires and uncontrolled sexual power (*shakti*) of their wives. Indeed, across South Asian contexts, unmet female desire is conceived of as a powerful force that has a tendency to spill over in excessive displays of mania, possession, or "hypomantic" states, as Gananath Obeysekere describes them.[28] According to the Indian psychoanalyst Sudhir Kakar's Jungian reading, archetypal Hindu femininity involves an inferior, dark side that is consistent with the forbidden desires that are incompatible with the strivings of the conscious persona. This shadow self is always there and must be managed, and at times released, so that it doesn't come to eclipse the persona.[29] Two symbolic models are often drawn on to frame such deviant or dangerous female desire in the Gaddi context—the witch and the wronged goddess Parvati. These models, while not dominant, were essential to representations of Gaddi femininity and framed whispers of *pagalpan*.

The witch (*dain*) is often framed as a woman whose aberrant desires come to inhabit and control her, causing her to engage in amoral, sexually transgressive, or antisocial behavior. "There are other languages, tantric mantras, that these witches know for doing something bad," another Gaddi companion explained. "They learn it from other witches, and so much fear comes from it. In modernity more people know these mantras, because there are more bad ideas and fewer good ideas in people's minds." Most often *dain* are widows or unmarried women who are uncontained by patriarchal structures of kinship. The performative, hypersexualized behavior that is associated with both *pagalpan* and witchcraft is written into Gaddi mythology, for instance, in retellings of the *dain maas*—an annual battle between witches and the god Indra Nag that occurs in the monsoon.[30] As Peter Phillimore writes, "The link between dains' power and their all-consuming sexuality emerges most strongly, in an annual battle they fight with the local gods atop a ridge of hills close to Karnathu, partly in Kangra and mostly in Mandi. This takes place at the start of Bhadron (August–September), and victory for the dains is achieved and symbolised by the sorceresses lifting up their dresses and taunting the gods (obliging the latter to withdraw)."[31]

Herein, symbolic formations of witchcraft and madness become entangled in models of deviant femininity that articulate what Nancy Munn has called the forms of "anti-value" that a society wishes to eschew or condemn.[32] The establishment of boundaries against witches or *pagal* women—through avoidance, emotional or physical violence leveled against them, or particular ritual practices—allows for the creation of a "protective separation rather than an expansion of connectivities," ultimately "counterposing oneself to the destructive other."[33] Yet these forms of anti-value remain potent, such that those who are associated with them hold a particular kind of agency or power.

A second symbolic model invoked in the understanding of madness can be found in the goddess Parvati. As Sarah Pinto describes, across India, Parvati is worshipped by Hindu women as the paragon of wifehood, a devoted consort of Lord Shiva, a domesticating, if passionate, female force.[34] However, Parvati's marriage is much more complicated than it seems on the surface. "Parvati," Wendy Doniger observes, "being a woman who places Kama [desire] foremost, cannot fathom the ascetic nature of the 'terrible' Shiva. She sees the mortal, domestic, superficial level . . . but is ignorant of the immortal, cosmic, inner level."[35] Parvati doesn't simply put up with the ascetic travails of her husband. Instead, quarrel, conflict, and discord abound in their marriage and are construed as an essential part of any sexual relationship, enhancing rather than impeding it.[36] Indeed, the unity of Shiva and Parvati is conceived as a cyclical symbolism—where Shiva quarrels with Parvati in his ascetic aspect and reunites with her in his erotic aspect.[37] This dynamic of unity and division is essential to Gaddi marriage. As we saw in the introduction, the story of Lord Shiva and Parvati for Gaddi people is not the representation of an abstract model for marriage, but marriage is considered a way of living *as* the divine couple.[38] In the Gaddi marriage ritual, the bridegroom disguises himself as a *jogi* (ascetic) prior to leaving for the bride's house. He is smeared in ash, clothed only in a lungi, and has flour *mundras* (*jogi*'s earrings) hung from his ears, a satchel slung over his shoulders, and a black *dora* (woolen rope) placed around his chest and wrists. He holds a begging bowl. In a performance in front of guests, he attempts to run away from the marital house and must be caught by his female kin—brought back into the folds of kinship and refocused on his marriage.

Parvati's story, as Pinto puts it, is one of "a woman in pieces, a shape shifter, constantly divided against herself, suffering in love and in the attempt to obtain her own freedom; her form speaking to the incompatible and uncomposed elements of womanhood."[39] It indicates the structural precarity of women in the marriage system, and the ambivalence of intimate relations that is carried by love. Neglect and violence are an important part of this blueprint. We see the goddess as a wife, always attempting to pull her husband back from his ascetic life, enticing him into the role of householder with her beauty and sexuality. Her inability to let her husband go as an ascetic is precisely what renders her weak and profane in comparison to her sacred and all-knowing husband. As such, in instances of madness, the marital cycle of quarrel and unity is broken, and women's sexual energy becomes dangerous and destructive. Like in the case of the witch, the uncontrolled sexual energy, while stigmatized, remains potent and powerful.

The symbolic models of both the witch and the goddess Parvati reveal other ways of thinking and being a woman that are otherwise unsayable. They are forms that exceed or escape the dominant symbolically constructed fantasies of domesticity and femininity. Mirroring the symbolic models of the witch and the wronged goddess, the narratives of *pagal* women like Shruthi and Tanu displayed contradictory, deviant behaviors that ran along the grooves of feminine ideals of care, motherhood, and housewifery but always seemed to spill over and go sprawling. These women were undone, often very publicly, forced to improvise in, to quote Clara Han, "normless experiments in life, where people engage to mitigate and normalize pains and distress at moments when these pains are problematized in everyday life."[40] They were seen in the eyes of the village to have failed as daughters, as mothers, as wives, and to have been failed by husbands, kin, and affines. They struggled to hold the lacunae of their own shame while they attempted to piece together their selfhood, to care for their children, and to love their husbands in new constellations. *Pagalpan* is a social process of stigmatization, but it is also a social process by which both a woman and the community around her acknowledge moments of relational impasse. At this impasse, women's unmet desires were seen as dangerous and powerful. While they faced acute exclusion and discrimination, *pagal* women were not abject subjects. Instead, they held an agency that issued from their deviant or unmet desires. I realized the full force of this when Pankaj came to visit me one bright April morning.

Pagaladevi Mata

Pankaj staggered up our stairs, clutching the railing, spittle dripping from his mouth. He stumbled onto the veranda and slumped against the wall of the house. Smriti, with whom I was sitting on the veranda, shot me a bemused look. Pankaj was always drunk. He haunted the small tea shops around the village, waiting for a drinking partner. One tended to cross the street to avoid his advances. Today was the first time he had come directly up to our house.

"My wife has left me." He wiped his nose on his shirt. "My wife and my children don't speak to me; it's because of my mother. This is why I drink." He stopped to slurp from the open bottle of Thums Up that he had filled with home-brewed desi spirits. "Please get me something to eat," he pleaded, attempting to salvage some kind of respectability by eating a small snack while drinking. "What can I do? All I can do is drink! My wife has become Pagaladevi Mata."

Again, he broke down, muttering something about how much he loved her. "These people have done some *jadu* on my wife," he cried out.

When I met Pankaj on that April day, he told me that it was shame (*sharam*) that led him to drink. He was ashamed by his wife's erratic behavior and sexual liaisons but also by his own culpability in driving her to madness, and his inability to protect her or meet her desires. To call her *pagal* was to admit that she was a victim of the precarity of a woman's position in marriage but could not be reintegrated back into kinship structures. To call her Pagaladevi Mata—the mad goddess—was to acknowledge the limit of her own human culpability and to register her excessive, destructive power.

THIS CHAPTER HAS BEEN concerned with extending the relational theory of distress that I have developed over the past four chapters to the question of madness. Doing so involves invoking a different point of departure in the study of madness from that which is usually taken in anthropological studies of severe mental illness. Rather than beginning spatially in the psychiatric clinic or the ritual healing shrine, I begin in the intimate, everyday relationships of a community in flux. Herein, I find madness not as a diagnostic category assigned by a psychiatrist but as a moral discourse that is the outcome of a fizz of rumor, speculation, and suspicion applied to people, and particularly to some who are unable to adjust to the vicissitudes of marriage. *Pagalpan*, as such, is generated through a social process of stigmatization that works to both exclude those who are considered deviant and acknowledge the trauma that they have experienced at the hands of intimate others who have failed them.

But the women who occupied these deviant social positionalities found something that, perhaps, their sisters and daughters who were less marginal did not have. The previous chapters have shown how *tension* allowed women to obliquely register and push back against the patriarchal, classed, and casted structures that did not serve them, while holding on to the fantasies of domesticity that sustained them. In this chapter we met women who were undone by their *tension*, who could no longer hold on to such fantasies, who directly critiqued or eschewed the structures that did not serve them. Such women provide models for an aesthetics of living otherwise. As an accused *pagal* woman, Shruthi shatters the fantasy of the good housewife by showing its contingency on fragile structures of marriage and kinship. Instead of adjusting, she attempted to take things into her own hands—seeking her own sexual gratification, earning her own money, seeking help from other men to get her jobs done. It was only by doing so that she could maintain what she thought was *izzat*. What made Shruthi *pagal* in the eyes of the village was that she was acting on her unmet desires. In doing so, she chose, clearly and visibly, to represent the conditions of her own suffering. As such, she offered an alternative way of living as an independent, albeit excluded woman, beyond the structures of alliance.

The kind of agency that comes with such deviance is thus not wholly resistant or directly political but something more experimental. It is characterized, as Andrew Lakoff puts it, by simulation, performance, in order to become something else.[41] The deviant behaviors of those considered *pagal* create a situation that breaks the familiar frame of perception. This works to introduce the uncanny into the fabric of the political world—where actions appear suspiciously political, and yet their explanation is not, subversive but not wholly antistructural. Displays of madness revealed an agonizing awareness of the precarity of women's condition within patriarchal kinship relations, rendered acute in the contemporary project of upward social mobility. *Pagal* women caused ripples of disturbance that amounted to no clear opposition of such patriarchal structures but issued from the contradictions of Gaddi marriage, mobilized the ambiguity of feminine tropes, and, as a result, remained aporetic to those around them. Their power was in mobilizing the inherent ambivalence of Gaddi femininity, rendering visible the simultaneous dependence on and disavowal of women in the upwardly mobile Gaddi community.

Coda

September 30, 2019

[5:20 a.m.] Smriti: Oh, you know they've moved out

[5:20 a.m.] Smriti: Long time ago

[5:20 a.m.] Nikita: Seriously

[5:21 a.m.] Nikita: To where?

[5:21 a.m.] Smriti: I probably forgot to tell you

[5:21 a.m.] Nikita: Pankaj too?

[5:21 a.m.] Smriti: They have been living in another village, on the other side of Dharamsala

[5:21 a.m.] Nikita: The whole family?

[5:21 a.m.] Smriti: No

[5:21 a.m.] Nikita: With another man or rented

[5:21 a.m.] Smriti: Only her and the kids

[5:21 a.m.] Nikita: What her daughters too?

[5:21 a.m.] Smriti: But her son came back to his grandmother

[5:22 a.m.] Smriti: The kids cried a lot

[5:22 a.m.] Nikita: Yeah god that's terrible to split them up

[5:22 a.m.] Nikita: Is she OK?

[5:22 a.m.] Smriti: They really miss their brother

[5:22 a.m.] Nikita: Where is Pankaj?

[5:22 a.m.] Smriti: He's still here I guess

Conclusion

CAN *TENSION* TRAVEL?

To Witness Is Not to Tell

This story of *tension* does not have an ending. Neither does the distress of the people that fill the pages of this book, nor my relational entanglements in and with this place.[1] As such, the careful narrative cuts that I make in writing this book are not organic, nor are they designed to give a sense of resolution. These narrative cuts—sometimes splices, sometimes excisions—are made to protect the anonymity of those who shared their *tension* with me, and to attempt, however inadequately, to hold and to render the waxing and waning of their distress. They are also made in cases where the relationships I had, and continue to have, exceeded the boundaries of research and became the stuff of our shared lives.

The beating heart of this book is to be found in the stories that I cannot tell you. These are stories—of illicit romance, abuse, violence, rape, incest, trauma, sexual yearning, pregnancy, hallucination, possession—that were told to me,

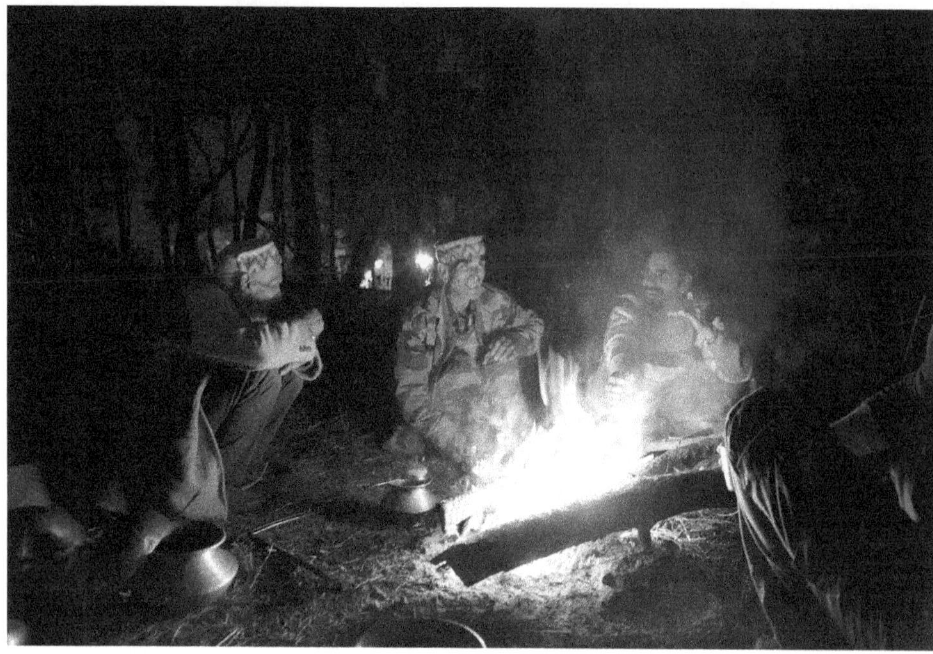

FIGURE C.1. Gaddi shepherds share stories by the *dera* (campsite). Photograph by Soujanyaa Boruah, 2024.

or that I witnessed, but that are not mine to relay. These are stories that sat heavily on my chest as I wrote and rewrote the ethnographic accounts herein. To witness distress is, as Deborah Thomas puts it, to attempt an "embodied practice." She writes, "It is a practice of recognition and love that destabilizes the boundaries between self and other, knowing and feeling, complicity and accountability. Witnessing . . . can therefore ultimately produce the internal shifts in consciousness that radiate from one to another in unexpected and necessarily nonlinear ways, and that lead to lasting, world-changing transformations."[2] For Thomas, witnessing is a form of embodied care that requires us to "recognize and respond to the psychic and sociopolitical dynamics in which we are complicit, and therefore to generate the ability to be response-able, to ourselves and to others."[3]

Being responsible for the stories of *tension* that I witnessed means that I cannot tell many of them. Instead, I do the only thing I feel that I can. I return to this place, and spend time with these people, year after year. I dance with them, eat with them, massage their aching backs, give them small gifts. I try my best to listen to how distress infuses their waking lives in new ways, propelling their relationships and haunting their dreams. I attend their weddings, and the weddings of their children. I attend the funerals of their fathers, and sometimes I attend their funerals. In being response-able, however, to the stories of *tension* that I witnessed, I hope that I have rendered a larger, fuller story of *tension* in this place—a story written against the violence of the many kinds of abstraction that sublimate distress.

A Slice of Time

Each time I return to the hills, I take the overnight bus from Majnu Ka Tilla in central Delhi. I get on as the sun is setting over the fetid Yamuna, and I close my eyes. I wake briefly in the early hours, my stomach lurching on impact with the Shivalik hills. In that time between sleep and waking, the sense of this place begins to fill me again. The warmth of the morning sun on my toes as I sit on the roof with Shankar. Iron digging into my finger joints as I cling to the back of a truck, hitching a ride down the main village road. As the bus winds around the last bends of Kangra town, the mountains rise. Each time, I see them anew, having forgotten the depth and majesty of the stage on which this story is set. The day has not quite started yet. The shops that line the road are still shut, and the air is cool. When I catch a glimpse of the wheat fields behind the road, I see heads bobbing and receding between the stalks. I look up from the golden fields to the scaly slate shore. I remember the slate wounds, cutting deeper each year into the mountains. Still caught by sleep, I lay my head back. I remember the mountains, how these great folds always leave something obscured from view. I imagine what lies behind those first ridges, on the other side of the crests and passes. Sometimes the range is lit up by the morning sun, but often, for months at a time, it is cloaked in heavy cloud. During the monsoon these fogs descend lower and lower, until they trickle into the valley and run through the houses. Here they meet the *tension* that has rolled in from the plains.

IN THIS BOOK I have attempted to capture the quick of this place as I encountered it. As the chapters of this book make clear, *tension* is not a signifier with a single meaning, nor is it a coherent condition, disease, or syndrome with clearly identifiable symptoms. Instead, the story of *tension* is a story of change—to the land, to the crops and weeds and flowers that grow on it, to livelihoods and the bodies that labor, to the gods and the souls that worship them. But most of all, it is a story of changing relationships between husbands and wives, parents and children, siblings, neighbors and friends, and even between people and their gods or ghosts. The Gaddi people whom you met in these pages talk about the psychic and embodied experience of such relational shifts as *tension*. In using this term, they do not separate out the "external" structural or relational tensions from these tensions' "internal" psychic or embodied effects. Instead, *tension* is a theory of distress that allows people to scale upward from their bodies, to feel out and to reshape their relations to intimate others and to the world around them.

This book puts forward *tension* as a gendered and relational theory of distress. It does not claim that it is new or necessarily innovative to think about mental distress as relational or gendered. As Keir Martin has shown, the psy-sciences and particularly psychotherapy—while accused of a preoccupation with the inner world—are more heterogeneous than their critics like to admit and hold within them elaborate models of relationality.[4] Indeed, anthropologists themselves have shown how psychologists, psychiatrists, and psychotherapists are deeply relational in their clinical and disciplinary encounters.[5] Despite this, these theories of gendered relationality still figure relationships as a property of the bounded individual, and the individual as mapped against networks of relationships. A deficit of relationships—in social isolation, stigma, or alienation—is said to result in mental ill health. As such, the antidote to mental ill health is often prescribed to be *more* relationships or *more* care.

The same individualism lives on in the way in which the psy-sciences think about the structural or social determinants of mental ill health. Herein, the "social" exists as a sphere or field that can be divided up into "factors" like housing, income, gender, or race that exist outside of an individual and come to "determine" their experience. The accounts in this book have shown several flaws in this view. First, this notion of the social is imprecise, as divisions between structural factors are empirically impossible and theoretically mystifying.[6] Second, individual experience is not determined by external social structures or relationships, but porous selves are constituted through these relationships. Third, relationships do not always issue positive affects. They generate distress as much as they heal it. Fourth, gender is not an idiosyncratic property of distress, but distress, or the question of who expresses it, experiences it, and absorbs it for others, is an instrument of patriarchy. To understand *tension* in particular and distress in general we must admit that sometimes, often even, relationships of care—however gendered—can cause exhaustion, anger, jealousy, and other negative affects. We understand these complex affects outside of a number of modernist distinctions that prevail in the psy-sciences: between the inside and the outside of the body, but also between the psyche and the soma and, even more fundamentally, between the bounded individual with desires and drives and the external social forces or even kinship relations that stand outside of them. Eschewing these distinctions, we come to think about the relational as an empirical question to be investigated. "It is in paying attention to the way relation is used," Marilyn Strathern writes, "that we might come closest to something like an ethnographic account of it."[7] This book, hence, is not a relational theory of distress everywhere but an account of a particular theory of gendered and relational distress held by and generated through a particular dynamic relational constellation of actors (humans, nonhumans, more-than-humans, and the environment) in a particular time. Even more specifically, it is generated through the subjective relational encounters that I had.

This book is a "slice of time" through which we might contend with the variable qualities and intensities of these relationships, in their presence and their absence.[8] We trace the stories, myths, symbols, and models through which people generate value from and ascribe meaning to these relationships. We watch them spin fantasies that structure and give consistency to the murk of experience. Within this slice of time, we find the forms of intimacy and mutuality that sustain the people of this place, and into which I was drawn. However, we also find the many misrecognitions, the forms of disconnection, of nonreciprocity and nonacknowledgment, of conflict and denial, that are inherent to any kind of relationality. These positive affects—joy, safety, well-being—are to be found in the moments where fantasies and aspirations are realized in and through the relationalities of life. We also watch as these fantasies and aspirations fail to be sustained by the care and acknowledgment of intimate others. In these moments, such fantasies fail to hold up in reality and they ferment into ambivalent or even painful affects and sensations—into envy, boredom, anger. They become lodged in the body as taut muscles, high blood pressure, wasting muscles, or aching joints. These bodies are, as Strathern puts it, "constructed as the plural and composite site of the relationships that produced them."[9] Both the proximate social and the generalized social are lived materially, or even anatomically, as forms of embodied subjectivity.[10] As such, fractures in relationships generate and are experienced as fractures in flesh and sinew, aches in head and heart.

Too often, the failure of acknowledgment or aspiration occurs for those who already experience a range of disadvantages and differences of sex, gender, caste, or class position. Indeed, power works *through* the deliberately unequal distribution of negative affects and sensations, like humiliation or exhaustion. Power, we might say, works through the unequal distribution of distress. However, this does not mean that those who absorb distress are powerless. The articulation of distress *does* something to renegotiate or resignify the unequal relational constellations that generate it. These acts of telling introduce a pause into the pulse of relations, allowing people who are oppressed by them to push back. Most of the time, as the preceding chapters have shown, this pushing back is subtle. It does not wholly resist or shatter relational constellations or reverse their inequalities. However, sometimes, as we saw in the final chapter, distress drives people to the edge of relations, leaving them with no choice but to seek alternative ways of living. These moments should not be glamorized, for they hold the most acute pain of exclusion, but from them emerges, sometimes, aesthetics of living otherwise.

IT TOOK ME A long time to realize that this "slice of time," and thus *tension*, cannot travel in the way that I wanted it to. Early in my fieldwork, as I was just starting to feel out the contours of *tension*, this question plagued me. For my anthropological insights to be relevant, I thought, *tension* had to be able to be found elsewhere as a cultural manifestation of a more natural, universal condition, or as a local manifestation of a global process.[11] The daughter and granddaughter of medical doctors, I sought constantly to extrapolate from multiple acts of telling *tension* to a wider condition of distress that might be recognizable in other contexts. I sought to taxonomize the symptoms that I listed during my interviews into neatly definable subconditions that could be associated with particular subgroups of this community—elderly people or lower-caste women, for example. Armed with experience working in global mental health, I also sought to associate this condition with various sociological processes or structural determinants of distress. Perhaps if my interlocutors were telling me that *tension* was new, it could be explained by some kind of broad, general force that could be found elsewhere. Perhaps it was caused by colonization, or urbanization, or sedentarization, or gentrification, or some layered and entangled abstraction of all of them.

However, when I listened again to the taped interviews that I had recorded, and when I sat with groups of women in creative workshops or over tea, their stories refused the abstractions that I tried to apply to them. Their symptoms slipped out of the categories and lists that I had allocated them to. When I returned from the field and began to organize these stories into chapters, the density of the ethnographic experiences that I had could not be tamed into a general disorder with subconditions that could be mapped onto specific groups. I realized that I couldn't call the slippery form of distress that my mother felt—nor any other form of distress I encountered elsewhere—*tension*, for these have different affects and are generated from different relational struggles.

Or if I did, the term *tension* would take on different qualities and meanings. It dawned on me that to apply either the abstraction of medical taxonomy or the abstraction of social or structural determinacy was a violence that would sublimate the relational qualities of the distress that was shared with me.

The will to abstract in this scientific way is part of a universalist, modernist epistemic project that is shared by the psy- and social sciences and embedded in different ways into questions of evidence, expertise, diagnostics, and treatment of mental illness. To describe mental disorders, as Michel Foucault showed us, is not a neutral act.[12] Instead, abstract psychiatric categories, shored up by the structures of scientific knowledge, are instruments of politics and governance that work through their power to define what is normative and what is not normative.[13] Many anthropologists have shown us how this works in situ through studies of psychiatric institutions and clinics, and more still have shown us how such categories take on new meanings or even ontologies in the flux of life.[14] However, the limited value placed on anthropological insights in hierarchies of scientific evidence mutes the potential for our discipline to "interfere," as João Biehl and Vincanne Adams put it, in the epistemic injustices that such abstractions perpetuate.[15] In policy, medical, and global health research, anthropology is often called on to offer "cultural" explanations for how a disease is manifesting, or why certain people aren't responding to treatment. Here, culture—like the relation—figures as a property of an individual rather than the individual being generated by and through culture. Part of the problem lies in the fact that medical anthropologists most often begin their studies of mental health in places where their interlocutors are already interpellated by therapeutic regimes (in psychiatric clinics or ritual healing shrines) before following their interlocutors into the spaces where most of life is lived (the domestic or neighborhood relations of care). This predetermines the forms of subjectivity that the researcher encounters. Anthropological accounts further parochialize themselves in the quest to render their insights intelligible to other disciplines—falling back on tools like the "cultural syndrome" or "idiom of distress," which are made to fit within medical epistemologies in order to uphold the distinction between nature and culture.

We also lose the clarity of our accounts when we scale up from distress, uncritically, to structural processes like colonialism, urbanization, or gentrification. The will to explain mental distress through such structural processes that somehow float above the murk of life is increasingly popular in economics and political science—seen most clearly in rising attention to "deaths of despair," as the Nobel Prize–winning economists Anne Case and Angus Deaton put it, and the rise of therapies like cognitive behavioral therapy and mindfulness

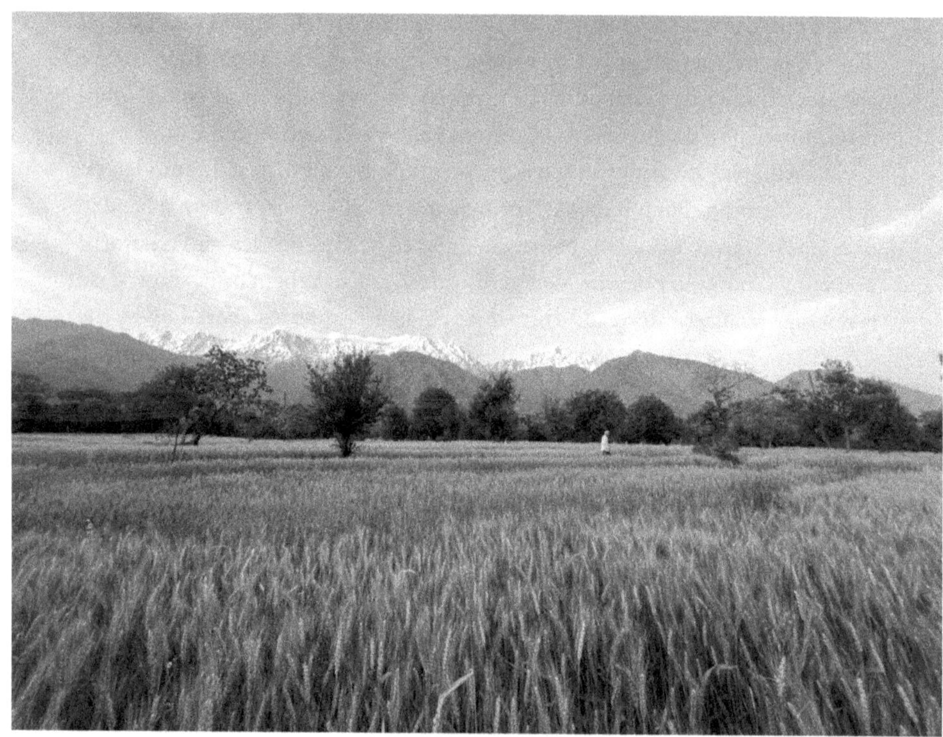

FIGURE C.2. Wheat fields in Kangra. Photograph by Nikita Kaur Simpson, 2023.

as remedies for the negative externalities of neoliberal austerity.[16] Likewise, environmental scientists are increasingly aware of the ways in which mental health renders visible the unequal effects of climate disaster—articulated in conditions like eco-anxiety, climate trauma, and ecological grief.[17] In both cases, the models of scale—between the distressed mind and these broader structural transformations—are heavy-handed and lack perspective on the "interscalar vehicles," as Gabrielle Hecht puts it, that people *themselves* use to scale between their bodies and wider forces.[18] The voices and theories of our interlocutors are hollowed out by these heavy-handed attempts at abstract scale—by the subsumption of the emic into the etic.

This book calls for a bolder anthropology of mental health, one that engages with but is not determined by the abstractions of medicine or psychiatry, of sociology or global health. For anthropological data and insights to be valuable in interdisciplinary research, policymaking, and clinical practice, they need not be universally applicable, scalable, or even replicable. Anthropologists are in a unique position to attend to the emic interscalar devices that our own interlocutors themselves generate, to speak to and critique wider changes. These might be emic moral categories, relational constellations, symbolic representations of the self, or bodily complaints. When we do so, the models of scale we find empirically often refuse linearity or verticality and force us to complicate the mechanisms of causality and responsibility that are implied in other disciplinary analyses. We bring into view forms of entanglement that resist and refuse modern liberal formations of nature, selfhood, embodiment, or the psyche. *Tension* acts as one of these interscalar vehicles whereby, through their disrupted bodies, people speak to the effects of colonial and state power and reflect on the limits of their agency in ways that complicate biomedical understandings of mental illness. This book has attempted to follow this interscalar vehicle along the pulsing relations of this place, not to fix it in place. I hope that it might inspire ever more nuanced and finely calibrated accounts of relationality and the way it generates distress.

Beyond Abstraction

But can *tension* travel? To answer this, we must return to a central problematic at the heart of the anthropological endeavor—the ethical and political implications of theorizing from ethnographic worlds. How do we do justice to emic theory without replicating problematic distinctions between the emic and the etic?[19] How do questions of ownership and authorship of theory become complicated in the scholarly publication process? How do we reconcile the importance of emic theory in a world where those who generate such theory receive little to no credit or material recompense, and those who render or translate it make careers?

The decolonizing ancestors of our discipline have argued for decades that the "researched" ought not to be subject to theory but ought to be credited as theorists themselves. More recently, Indigenous scholars have renewed the call for anthropologists to, in the words of Métis scholar Zoe Todd, "[credit Indigenous peoples] as thinkers in their own right, not just disembodied representatives of an amorphous Indigeneity that serves European intellectual or political purposes, and not just as research subjects or vaguely defined 'collaborators.'"[20] This book has attempted to respond to Todd's call by providing a platform for the Gaddi theory of distress as a theory that might speak back to both Western psychiatry and social science. Herein, I am not arguing that *tension* cannot travel at all but that it ought not travel by being subsumed in a Western medical taxonomy or model of structural force. Instead, it ought to travel on its own terms, with the appropriate credit for the nuanced depictions of scale and relationality, affect and embodiment, that it holds. It ought to be pitched against universalizing models of distress and be used to reveal their contingencies and provincialize their dominant assumptions. And when it does travel—as it already has and surely will resonate with experiences of fraught relationality, distress, and change elsewhere—it will hopefully allow others to name and even feel sensations and experiences that are otherwise unnameable or unfeelable, as it did for me when I reflected back on the *tension* that I encountered in my mother's body. As such, it will not travel as a neat abstraction but become a new kind of "situated knowledge," in Donna Haraway's terms, taking on other projects, affects, fantasies, and relationalities, and thus be forever changed.[21] This does not answer the question of "credit" that Todd poses. This scholarly publication will do little for the theorists of *tension* whom I met. Here I turn to other creative forms of research creation—devised with my interlocutors and developed over years—to generate intergenerational conversations, spaces for artistic creation and activism, and "fugitive" practices that allow me to remain response-able to my collaborators.

To this end, I conclude by inviting you to experiment with *tension* through a different form of language, the notation of dance and movement scores. A score is a form of notation that shows a sequence of movements that a dancer might use.[22] For me, experimenting with movement scores has allowed me to feel out—affectively, atmospherically, and corporeally—experiences of *tension* beyond the empirical formulations that I encountered. What I felt in devising such scores, and what others (students, friends, colleagues) have felt in performing them, has resonated with, but is different from, what my interlocutors felt. Perhaps in engaging with this score you will come to feel *tension* in a particular, situated way. Consider and perhaps try the following example, or devise your own:

Put down this book and sit up straight.
Release your shoulder blades down your back.
Ground your feet to the floor and feel your soles pushing up into your hips.
Set your gaze straight and close your eyes.
Now pull your jaw back and constrict the muscles in the back of your neck.
Feel the constriction at the base of your skull.
Release.
Do it again.
Notice how the heat pools in the back of your head.
Notice how the frequency resonates in other parts of your body.

Acknowledgments

The pages of this book are but an imprint of the rich web of relations that have made it.

The seeds for this project were planted in two places: first, in the Anthropology Department at the University of Cambridge, and particularly in a conversation with Perveez Mody on my return from undergraduate fieldwork in the Himalayas that exceeded our allocated supervision time by some hours; and, second, in the creative environment created by Anna Kydd at the SHM Foundation, where I first encountered the emergent worlds of global mental health and learned from the Khuluma mentors.

These seeds grew in a vibrant doctoral program at the London School of Economics (LSE), with thanks to the incredible teaching and support of the Anthropology Department. I give special thanks to Deborah James, Catherine Allerton, Mukulika Banerjee, Jonny Parry, Nick Long, Luke Heslop, and the late David Graeber for watering these seeds. My doctoral cohort was and continues to be extraordinary. I have learned so much from each one of them: Sam Wilby, Megan Rose Donnelly, Arturo Gonzales, Ignacio Sandoval, Imani Strong, Hannah Cottrell, Agathe Faure, Pengyin Kong, Jaskiran Kaur, Jonathan Doherty, Kite Tengparwat, and Angela Giattino. Deep friendships from the LSE also made this book during my postdoc, including with the Doctors Without Books group and the Covid and Care Research Group. Yan Hinrichsen's support has been invaluable. Megnaa Mehtta, Giulio Ongaro, Michael Edwards, Megan Laws, and Andrea Pia have been inspirational companions.

At the LSE, this research was generously supported by an LSE PhD studentship (2016–20). Fieldwork was made possible by a Fredrick Williamson Memorial Fund Grant (2014) in the preliminary stages and by the Alfred Gell Research

Proposal Prize (2017) in later stages. The writing-up process was supported by the Raymond and Rosemary Firth Award (2020–21). The LSE Department of Anthropology also supported language and mental health counseling training.

This project has been shepherded by two formidable scholars. Alpa Shah's unwavering support is the backbone of this book. Laura Bear's creativity and courage is its heart. You will find my attempt to take forward their legacies in this book, however inadequate. They encourage me to dwell in the nuance of life, and I am a better ethnographer, and hopefully a better person, for it.

At the School of Oriental and African Studies (SOAS), this manuscript has come into being through the generosity and support of colleagues in the Anthropology Department. The school also provided a Research Culture Fund Award (2023–24) to develop this into a book manuscript. I give particular thanks to Emma Crewe, Catherine Dolan, Ed Simpson, and Marloes Janson for inviting me into the department; to Alice Rudge and Saad Quasem for drawing out ecological implications of my work; and to my colleagues at the Centre for Anthropology and Mental Health Research in Action (CAMHRA), Michelle Callander, Fabio Gygi, Naomi Leite, Orkideh Behrouzan, Neil Armstrong, and Bhrigupati Singh, for encouraging me to be much more ambitious with the arguments I make. David Mosse's wisdom guides me each day. It is the greatest honor to journey beside you all into this next phase of CAMHRA work.

Beyond my institutional homes, this book has benefited from intellectual exchanges across the world. Some of the most fruitful exchanges have been with Megan Moodie, Cynthia Ling Lee, Marina Peterson and the University of California Humanities Research Institute Long Hauling collective, Tine Gammeltoft, Richard Rechtman, Jane Dyson, Craig Jeffrey, Sophie Chao, Tim Cooper, Elizabeth Storer, Suad Duale, Mardi Reardon-Smith, and Marilyn Strathern. Thank you for listening to me.

This project builds on a deep history of scholarship with and about Gaddi life. My greatest joys have been engaging particularly with Peter Phillimore, Christina Noble, Rich Axelby, and Kriti Kapila—sharing photographs, stories, myths, artifacts. I also build on the work of Anya Wagner, Minoti Chakravarty-Kaul, Stephen Christopher, and many others.

This manuscript has been honed by the sharp eyes of two anonymous reviewers, as well as the encouraging words of many who have reviewed unpolished drafts and article-length manuscripts. It was turned from stodgy prose to story through the magic of James Moran. I am deeply grateful to Ken Wissoker for taking a chance on me, and to both Ken and Kate Mullen for their editorial support.

In India, this fieldwork was made possible through the institutional support of Jawaharlal Nehru University and South Asian University in Delhi. I particularly thank Ankur Datta for paving the first steps for me. To Niki, Pravir, Anup, Malli, Ruchi Masi, Preeti Masi, Dimple Masi—I will forever cherish the time I was able to spend with you. I can't imagine what it will be like to return without Veerji Nana and Didi Nanni and have deep gratitude that I was able to spend time with them where my own mother and Nanni could not. Thank you to Neelu and Teji, who kept that annex for me (and for the beautiful photographs, also featured here). To my friends—Shantu, Nimisha, Gauri, Rhea, Rahul, and all your gang—thank you for giving me the break I needed from deeply sad stories in your Green Park rooftop.

In Dharamsala, I was welcomed by Colonel Bhagat, Kindhi, and Basu. I was led to the bucolic foothills of the Dhaula Dhar by the kindness of Kirin Narayan and Ken George. There I met so many who steadied me—thanks to Hannah Carlan, the late Didi Contractor, Maya Narayan, Kishwar Shirali, Edith Stein, and Barbara Nath Wiser. I am so grateful to have been able to use the Nishta space for workshops and to draw on your invaluable insights on the village. Thanks to the friends I made in the village—Rony, Prasenjit, Ishaan, Aditi, Asanda, and Anish especially—and the friends from far away who came to visit me there. There are many in this place whom I can't name but to whom this book is indebted.

I would have been wandering around aimlessly for a year if it hadn't been for Soujanyaa and Shyam, who found me. It is to them that I owe this project, though all errors remain mine. Another version of this book is an epic of our many adventures together, and of your love story. This book is also indebted to Shyam's family—to Aunty, Saroj Didi, Mohinder Jiju, Gugli, RB, KB, Bony Jiju, and most of all Vandu Didi (and Dakshu and Eva).

Finally, to my own family: This is a piece of writing, above all, about the strains and joys of loving your kin.

To Iona and Archie for being my family in Peckham.

To Tony and Nicola for being there in the hardest times.

To my grandparents—Judy, David, Avtar, and Prithi—whose journeys inspired me to leave the shelters of home.

To my siblings—Rohan, Saachin, and Maya—for pulling me back to earth.

To my parents—Rani and Ian—for never, ever failing to support me. I love you all the rice.

To Hugo, *meri jaan*, who has followed me around the world, I am always at home with you.

Select Hindi and Gaddi Glossary

Adjust karna parega (एडजस्ट करना पड़ेगा): Adjust
Asrat (असरात): An effect
Atta-satta (अत्ता-सत्ता): Exchange marriage
Azadi (आज़ादी): Individual freedom
Baat (बात): Happenings
Berry (बेरी): Anger toward a lover
Bhava (भाव): A shared mood
Bhiog (भोग): Grief, particularly for a lover or partner
Bhut (भूत): Ghost
Bimar (बमिार): Sick, ill
Bojh (बोझ): Pressure, burden
BP (बीपी): High or low blood pressure, often undiagnosed
Cela (सेला): Ritual healer
Churel (चुरैल): Ghosts of women who were infertile or died in childbirth
Dagi (डागी): Male witch
Dain (डाइन): Female witch
Dain maas (डाइन मास): Annual battle between witches and Indra Nag
Dan-pan (दान-पन): Marriage by gift
Dant-band (दांत-बंद): A psychological condition where the jaw becomes locked
Den/dain (डेन/डाइन): A term for witch
Deopuchna (देवपूछना): Afflictions
Dera (डेरा): Campsite or campfire
Devi-devta (देवी-देवता): Gods and goddesses
Dhar (धार): Shepherding hut, alpine pastures
Dharam (धर्म): Moral way of life seated in place, community, work, and landscape
Dhundu (धुंडू): Gaddi name for Lord Shiva
Dimagi (दमिागी): Mind
Dimagi ki problem (दमिागी की प्रॉब्लम): Problem of the mind
Dogar (डोगर): Wizard
Dora (डोरा): Woolen rope

Ghabrahat, dil ka ghabrahat (घबराहट, दलि का घबराहट): Panic attack, heart palpitations
Ghar ka kaam (घर का काम): Housework
Ghar ki (घर की): Household (as in household worries)
Ghoonghat (घूंघट): Veiling of women in front of their male relatives and sexual avoidance
Ghum (ग़म): Sorrow or sadness
Gorji (गोर्जी): Gaddi name for Parvati
Guttan (गुट्टन): A sense of suffocation, like that in panic or anxiety
Ilaaj (इलाज): Ritual or treatment
Izzat (इज्जत): Honor, respectability
Jadu, or jadu tona (जादु, या जादू टोना): Witchcraft
Jana (जना): Tribe
Jati (जाती): Caste
Jogi (जोगी): Ascetic
Jogni (जोगनी): A term for witch
Kaam (काम): Work, labor
Kajal (काजल): Eyeliner
Kali yug (कली युग): The fourth stage in the repeating cycle of increasing moral decay in Hindu cosmology
Kamzor (कमज़ोर): Weak (noun)
Kamzori (कमज़ोर): Weak (adj.)
Karewa (करेवा): Widow's remarriage
Kul devis (कुल देवी): Clan-based goddesses of the home
Lambardhars (लम्बरदार): Landowners
Mahaul (माहौल): Atmosphere
Malhundi (मलहुंडी): The head of the flock
Mata aye (माता आई): Possession by a goddess
Maya (माया): Relational and physical net, said to be illusory, also referred to as "Moh-Maya"
Mirgi (मरि्गी): Epilepsy
Najaiz faida (नाजायज़ फ़ायदा): Abuse
Nazar (नज़र): Evil eye
Nuala (नुअला): Shaivite ritual that includes a goat sacrifice
Opara (ओपारा): Black magic
Pagal (पागल): Mad
Pagalpan (पागलपन): Madness
Paghiri (पघीरी): Bonded laborers
Pani ki problem (पानी की समस्या): Vaginal discharge
Piliya (पीलिया): Jaundice
Prem (प्रेम): Love
Purvaj (पूर्वज): Ancestors
Ras (रस): Juices or essences in the body
Rog (रोग): Physical illness
Sadhu (साधु): Renouncer, ascetic
Sasural (ससुराल): Husband's village

Shakti (सक्ती): Libidinal life force
Shaq (शक): Doubt
Sharabi (शराबी): An alcoholic
Sharam (शर्म): Shame
Samay (समय): The burden of time and life events
Sariri (सारीरी): Natural
Shamlat (शमलात): Communal or waste land
Shanth (शांत): Peaceful
Sindoor (सिंदूर): Vermilion
Sukh-dukh (सुख-दुःख): Ups and downs in life
Tanav (तनाव): Tension, stress, strain
Takat (ताकत): Physical strength
Tension ki bimari (टेंशन की बीमारी): Tension sickness
Warisi (वारसी): Grant from Raja to use grazing land
Zamana (ज़माना): The times we live in

Notes

INTRODUCTION

1. For a full account of this ritual, see Phillimore, "Marriage and Social Organisation," 308–9.

2. Hunter, *Imperial Gazetteer*, 301–2.

3. Hunter, *Imperial Gazetteer*, 301–2.

4. See Narayan, *Mondays*.

5. See Govindrajan, "Labors of Love," 199.

6. Wadley, *Shakti*.

7. Kapila, "Measure of a Tribe."

8. Xaxa, *State, Society and Tribes*, 1–2.

9. Kapila, "Measure of a Tribe"; Christopher, "'Scheduled Tribe Dalit.'" As Kriti Kapila suggests, the watershed was the Mandal Commission's recommendations in the 1990s that positive discrimination should be extended not only to the ritually and/or "civilizationally" deprived sections of India but also to what were termed "economically backward classes." Gaddi Rajputs, Thakurs, and Ranas were adamant that they would not be classified as Other Backward Classes but sought recognition as ST for their distinctive way of life.

10. Kapila, "Measure of a Tribe."

11. See Tilche, *Adivasi Art*; and Simpson, "Aesthetic Politics."

12. I use the term *lower-caste* as opposed to *dalit* as the latter term was not widely used during my time of fieldwork.

13. Hota, *Violence of Recognition*, 4.

14. Xaxa, *State, Society and Tribes*, 15.

15. Xaxa, *State, Society and Tribes*, 3.

16. This project of respectability is only partly attributable to Hindu nationalist ideology. Unlike neighboring Uttarakhand, Himachal Pradesh is predominantly Hindu but does not have a deep history of Hindutva grassroots activism, and Gaddi people support both the ruling Bharatiya Janata Party (BJP) and the Indian Congress Party (ICP).

17. Pinney, "Living in the Kal(i)yug."

18. Ngai, *Ugly Feelings*, 14.

19. Rutherford, "Affect Theory."

20. V. Das, *Life and Words*, 8.

21. V. Das, *Life and Words*, 216.

22. See Martin, *Psychotherapy, Anthropology*, for an in-depth analysis of interiority and exteriority in psychology.

23. Schnegg, "Collective Loneliness." Schnegg draws on the work of phenomenologist Hermann Schmitz and feminist theorist Sarah Ahmed.

24. Gammeltoft, "Domestic Moods," 10.

25. B. Singh and Sharan, "Contagion." Herein *tension* is akin to the *asrat* in some instances that Bhrigupati Singh and Pratap Sharan write of; see chapter 5.

26. GD Mental Disorders Collaborators, "Burden."

27. Arias et al., "Quantifying Global Burden."

28. Qureshi, *Chronic Illness*, 123; J. Das et al., "Mental Health Gender-Gap"; Weaver, "Tension Among Women"; Weaver, *Sugar and Tension*. Anthropologists and community psychologists have begun to draw out the relational meanings of *tension*, seeing it as the embodied and psychologically internalized stress of supporting kin in conditions of scarcity. *Tension* is seen as serving a communicative purpose, expressing dissatisfaction with life and difficulties in fulfilling social roles, and allowing the sufferer to seek outside help. Yet none of these studies, except for Weaver's ("Tension Among Women"; *Sugar and Tension*), look at *tension* on its own terms, instead seeing it alongside a range of other chronic illnesses or idioms of distress. Beyond the Indian context, see Wardell, *Living in the Tension*.

29. Ramaswami, "Masculinity"; Halliburton, "'Just Some Spirits.'"

30. V. Das, *Affliction*; Grover, *Marriage, Love, Caste*; Atal and Foster, "'Life Is Tension.'"

31. Weaver, "Tension Among Women," 44.

32. Govindrajan, "Labors of Love," 199.

33. While the presence of Hindutva activist organizations in Himachal Pradesh is comparatively less than in neighboring states, Daniela Berti notes the efforts of the Akhil Bharatiya Itihas Sankalan Yojana (ABISY) in Kangra as focused on resignifying the region's name and history. She writes, "In the district of Kangra, south-east of Himachal Pradesh, the unit's project deals with Trigarta, an ancient name for this area. One ABISY publication entitled Yug-yugin trigarta (Trigarta through the ages) translates Trigarta as 'three valleys' which, as explained in the Foreword, would correspond to a 'distinct socio-cultural and political entity, [whose] history goes back to before Mahabharata.'" Berti, "Local Enactment of Hindutva," 68.

34. See Bessire, *Behold the Black Caiman*; and Chao, *In the Shadow*. I have found it particularly helpful to compare *tension* to the *abu abu* that Sophie Chao recounts as affecting the Marind people of Merauke in West Papua, and the Black Caiman that affects the Ayoreo of the Gran Chaco—where rapid incursions of capitalist development are shaping the psychic and embodied worlds of Indigenous people.

35. Gaddi people do not use either the term *Indigenous* or the term *Adivasi* to describe their claim to custodianship of land. See Eubanks and Sherpa, "We Are," for a deeper discussion of Indigenous social movements in India.

36. *Oxford English Dictionary*, "tension," accessed July 18, 2025, https://www.oed.com/dictionary/tension_v.

37. Hydraulic models of blood pressure and *tension* are also described in Cohen, "Anthropology of Senility"; and V. Das, *Affliction.*

38. Crocq, "History of Anxiety."

39. Jadhav, "Western Depression," 278.

40. Rabinbach, *Human Motor*, 51, quoted in Jadhav, "Western Depression."

41. Rabinbach, *Human Motor*, 153.

42. Marx, quoted in Blackledge, *Marxism and Ethics*, 50.

43. Jadhav, "Western Depression."

44. See Jadhav, "Western Depression," 279.

45. Venkat, *Limits of Cure*, 39.

46. Arnold, *Colonizing the Body*; Stoler, "Making Empire Respectable"; Bear, *Lines of the Nation.*

47. Venkat, *Limits of Cure*, 38.

48. Venkat, *Limits of Cure*, 39.

49. Fanon, *Wretched of the Earth*, 53.

50. Fanon, quoted in Scott, *Extravagant Abjection*, 40.

51. Scott, *Extravagant Abjection*, 48.

52. Scott, *Extravagant Abjection*, 65.

53. See Delvecchio-Good et al., *Postcolonial Disorders.*

54. Nichter, "Idioms of Distress."

55. Ravi N. Singh, personal communication, November 2024.

56. Jadhav, "Western Depression."

57. Wilson, *Gut Feminism.*

58. Biehl and Moran-Thomas, "Symptoms."

59. Patel and Oomman, "Mental Health Matters Too"; Rodrigues et al., "Listening to Mothers"; Kermode et al., "Empowerment of Women"; Paralikar et al., "Cultural Epidemiology."

60. Patel et al., "Poverty."

61. Shidhaye and Patel, "Socio-Economic, Gender and Health Factors"; T. Roberts et al., "Is There a Medicine?"

62. B. Singh, "Can a Neighborhood Fall Sick?"

63. The "cultural syndrome" approach was developed by Byron Good, looking at heart distress in Iran. A cultural syndrome indicates "typical experiences, a set of words, experiences and feelings, which 'run together' for the members of a society." Good, "Heart," 26–27. An idiom of distress is an evolving set of specific words, phrases, and even actions that people use in different cultural contexts to express and respond to distress. Nichter, "Idioms of Distress." See also Nichter, "Idioms of Distress Revisited"; and Kaiser and Weaver, "Culture-Bound Syndromes," for an updated analysis of how to use idioms of distress in ways that take into account interpersonal, structural, and symbolic dynamics.

64. Kleinman, "Anthropology and Psychiatry," 452.

65. Tsing et al., "Patchy Anthropocene."

66. Agard-Jones, "Bodies," 192.

67. Campt, *Listening to Images*, 26, 54. Campt uses the example of passport photographs of Ugandan migrants to Birmingham. She encourages us to pay attention to

"these sublimely quiet images" as they "enunciate an aspirational politics that are accessible at the lowest of frequencies" (26).

68. Gilroy, *Black Atlantic*, 37.

1. *OPARA*

Some of the ethnographic accounts and analysis in this chapter also appear in Nikita Simpson, "Encountering the Dain," *HIMALAYA: The Journal of the Association for Nepal and Himalayan Studies* 42, no. 2 (2023): 70–85.

1. Bear, "Doubt, Conflict, Mediation," 9.
2. See Cooper et al., "Back/s to the Present."
3. Berlant, *Cruel Optimism*, 4.
4. Xaxa, *State, Society and Tribes*, 14.
5. Kapila, "Governing Morals."
6. See Dirks, *Castes of Mind.*
7. Kapila, "Governing Morals," 19.
8. Christopher and Phillimore, "Exploring Gaddi Pluralities," 7.
9. Christopher and Phillimore, "Exploring Gaddi Pluralities," 7.
10. Lyall, *Report*, 32, 47–48. Lyall writes, "The right to collect the grazing fees paid by Gaddi shepherds was at first transferred to the communities, but the shepherds at once objected, and showed that the measure would injure them, as the boundaries of their runs did not coincide with the boundaries of the mauzalis; so Mr. Barnes, with the sanction of the Chief Commissioner, annulled the transfer. The same objection did not apply in the case of, the dues or rent hitherto paid to the State by other persons, such as the Giijar herdsmen, the quarriers, iron-smelters, netters of falcons, owners of water-mill" (xii).
11. Lyall, *Report*, 46.
12. In relation to religion, Gaddis were recorded in the census of 1901 as of the same pastoralist group as Muslim Gadis of Karnal and Delhi. This was corrected in 1911, when the two groups were separated on religious grounds—where the Gaddis of the hills were noted for their Hindu beliefs, as opposed to the Muslim Gadis of the plains. The Gaddis were also distinguished from Muslim Gujjar buffalo herders who inhabit the hills and, often, the same pastures. For analysis of Gaddi-Gujjar relations from colonial times to the present, see Kapila, "Governing Morals," 48; and Axelby, "'Who Has the Stick.'"
13. Barnes, *Report*, 154–55.
14. Skaria, "Shades of Wildness"; Skaria, "Women, Witchcraft."
15. Rose, *Tribes and Castes*, iii.
16. Rose, *Tribes and Castes*, i.
17. Xaxa, *State, Society and Tribes*, 15.
18. Kapila, "Governing Morals," 72.
19. Sharabi, "Politics of Madness," 186.
20. Pinney, "Living in the Kal(i)yug," 78.
21. In November 2016 the Indian national government announced that they would render all five hundred– and thousand-rupee notes obsolete and issue new notes. This

was aimed at curtailing the cash economy in India, promoting electronic banking and payments, and regulating taxation.

22. Sharma, "Symbols of Empowerment"; Sharma, "Ritual, Performance and Transmission."

23. Punjab Government, *States Gazetteer of Chamba*, 203. Oral histories suggest that the shepherding economy was organized historically such that primarily Rajputs, including Khatris, Ranas, and Thakurs, engaged in shepherding. In some instances, Gaddi-speaking Brahmins also kept herds. Not all Gaddis engaged in shepherding or had their own flocks; evidence suggests that some Gaddis threshed rice or worked in the homes of others during the winter months in Kangra. Punjab Government, *States Gazetteer of Chamba*, 203. Some shepherds were also hired by wealthy peasants in the plains to keep flocks. Lower-caste Halis and Sipis were often employed as agricultural laborers or as waged servants to shepherds—where they were provided lodging, food, and shoes.

24. C. Singh, *Natural Premises*, 17; Kapila, "Governing Morals," 17.

25. Saberwal, *Pastoral Politics*; Kapila, "Governing Morals."

26. Bhattacharya, "Pastoralists"; Kapila, "Governing Morals."

27. Punjab Government, *Gazetteer of the Kangra District* (1885), 127.

28. Kapila, "Governing Morals," 20; Christopher, "'Scheduled Tribe Dalit'"; Chowdhry, *Veiled Women*.

29. Axelby, "'It Takes Two Hands,'" 69.

30. Ahmead, *Khanayara Stone Quarries*.

31. The economic structure of the industry was unique, as it privileged the communities in which the mines were set. When the "Company," for instance, stopped paying revenues to the villagers, the Khagota Panchayat took the Company to the Lahore High Court, which ruled such nonpayment illegal.

32. Axelby, "'Who Has the Stick.'"

33. Christopher, "'Scheduled Tribe Dalit,'" 7–8. Christopher writes, "Shepherding families now take Hali servants (*nokar*) from Chamba or non-Gaddi helpers from Panjab or Rajasthan and foster their own trajectory to owning flocks. However, SCs are barred from official shepherding associations, crucial institutions to regional electoral politics, such as the Gaddi Welfare Board and Wool Federation."

34. Kapila, "Measure of a Tribe," 124.

35. Christopher, "'Scheduled Tribe Dalit'"; Kapila, "Measure of a Tribe."

36. Christopher, "'Scheduled Tribe Dalit.'"

37. Bear, *Lines of the Nation*; Shah and Lerche, *Ground Down by Growth*; Parry, *Classes of Labour*.

38. N. Roberts, *To Be Cared For*.

39. Mosse et al., "Minds of Caste."

40. Guru, *Humiliation*.

41. As Nate Roberts shows in the case of the Pariyar caste. N. Roberts, *To Be Cared For*.

42. Mosse et al., "Minds of Caste," 1.

43. One of the most acute and common manifestations of *opara* was spirit possession. Possession by the goddess Kali (sometimes as her general form and sometimes as specific

manifestations), by *kul devta* or *devi* (household god or goddess), or by malign spirits like ghosts (*bhut*) is a common occurrence for all Gaddis but particularly for women at liminal stages of the life course, like just before marriage or during pregnancy, occurring both spontaneously in the flux of daily life, during ritual prayers and festivals, or when called by a *cela* in therapeutic settings. As Asaf Sharabi notes elsewhere in Himachal Pradesh, the distinction between the possession states of institutionalized ritual specialists and laypeople is not clear-cut in the Gaddi context. Sharabi, "Politics of Madness." Those who have "weak minds," caused by illness, previous affliction by *opara*, or lack of intelligence, are prone to possession. It is said that the "mata comes" (*mata aye*) to "play" with the possessed (*khelna*). The afflicted sometimes experience a "displacement of the self," lose their sense of conscious reality, and perform all manner of erratic movements, which they will not remember after the Mata leaves them. When the Mata comes, the person is treated as if they embody the Mata herself, where those around them bow and pray in her presence, muttering *jai mata*. This viewing of the god is referred to as *darśan*; see Sharabi, "Politics of Madness." Such possession has a variety of meanings, sometimes situational and sometimes therapeutic. However, it is often used as a therapeutic mechanism by ritual healers (*cela or celi*) to cure or correct afflicted people from illness or the curse of *jadu*. The Mata will possess the *cela*, who will go into trance, during which they will relay the wishes of the Mata in her voice. This is usually a vague and nonspecific description of who or what has caused the affliction, and a prescription of the kind of actions, restrictions, and avoidances that the afflicted must undergo in order to shore up the boundaries of the body and be rid of the malign force. For more detail on Gaddi spirit possession, see Sharma, "Symbols of Empowerment"; and Christopher, "Black Magic"; and for more detail on possession in the Himalayas, see Sax, *God of Justice*; Sharabi, "Politics of Madness"; and Berti, "Possession, Communication."

44. See Sharabi, "Politics of Madness." It is important to note, however, that local *devi-devta* (gods and goddesses) didn't play as large a role in Gaddi everyday life and politics as they seem to in ethnographic analyses of the nearby Kullu, Garhwal, and Parvati valleys, perhaps because of Gaddi Shaivite animistic religiosity and stronger ritual links to Chamba. They don't, for example, perform *devtā kā rāj* (government by deity).

45. Bindi, "Denouncing."

46. Berti, "Possession, Communication," 1–2.

47. Ngai, *Ugly Feelings*, 1.

48. Pollock, quoted in Khera, *Place of Many Moods*, 13.

49. Khera, *Place of Many Moods*, 12.

50. As Geoffrey Hughes and colleagues have put it, negative emotional states of others, and especially envy, can be "physically deleterious" to oneself. These emotions encode themselves through elaborate ethnophysiologies of contagion, often framed as forms of witchcraft. Hughes et al., "Introduction."

51. Particular clan groups within the Gaddi castes, such as the Mogu clan, had a reputation for their knowledge of tantric practices. Most of the men considered to practice witchcraft were from the Mogu clan and labeled *dagi*.

52. Phillimore, "'Famous Village,'" 176. As Helen Macdonald reflects in her monograph on witchcraft in Chhattisgarh, the revelation of witchcraft in a contemporary

world often involves a slow and fragmentary process of attunement to the subversive economy of rumor and suspicion. Macdonald, *Witchcraft Accusations.*

53. Munn, *Fame of Gawa*, 219–26.

54. There is a wealth of literature on witchcraft and other uncanny figures as the dark underbelly of social relations. See particularly Geschiere, *Modernity of Witchcraft*; Bubandt, *Empty Seashell*; and Ashforth, *Witchcraft, Violence, and Democracy*.

55. Bubandt, *Empty Seashell*, xvi, 32.

56. Bubandt, *Empty Seashell*, 32.

57. Bubandt, *Empty Seashell*, xvi.

58. Here I follow Bear and colleagues, who extend Munn's argument about how socially generative time works; Munn emphasizes the labor of time that people are involved in. "We argue that the act of working in and on time involves: an encounter with the material world; the limits of the body; multiple tools; and co-ordinations of diverse rhythms and representations." Bear, "Doubt, Conflict, Mediation," 20.

59. Marsilli-Vargas, *Genres of Listening*, 4.

60. E. V. Daniel, *Fluid Signs*, 109; see also Trawick, *Love in a Tamil Family*. It is through the control of the substances and moods of the house, and the substances and sentiments of the (gendered) body, that communities establish their boundaries and maintain the purity of their lineage.

61. Lamb, "Making and Unmaking"; see also Marriott, *Hindu Transactions*.

62. For a discussion of the "bio-moral," see Bear, *Lines of the Nation*.

63. Geschiere, "Witchcraft."

64. Scarry, *Body in Pain*, 3–4.

65. Scarry, *Body in Pain*, 13.

66. Denyer Willis, "In Attention to Pain," 357.

2. *KAMZORI*

An earlier version of this chapter appears in Nikita Simpson, "*Kamzori*: Aging, Care and Alienation in the Post-Pastoral Himalaya," *Medical Anthropology Quarterly* 36, no. 3 (2022): 391–411.

1. See Wagner, *Gaddi Beyond Pastoralism*, 44 (for a description of marriage celebrations).

2. Cohen, "Anthropology of Senility"; Cohen, *No Aging in India*; Snell-Rood, *No One*; V. Das, *Affliction*; Weaver, "Tension Among Women."

3. Marriott, "Female Family Core"; Marriott, *Hindu Transactions*; Lamb, "Making and Unmaking"; Lamb, *White Saris*.

4. Lamb, *White Saris*, 147.

5. Wadley, "No Longer a Wife."

6. Deleuze, "Active and Reactive," quoted in B. Singh, "Anthropological Investigations of Vitality," 550.

7. Singh, "Anthropological Investigations of Vitality."

8. Singh, "Anthropological Investigations of Vitality," 558.

9. *Kaam* has no particular etymological relation to *kamzori*.

10. Axelby, "'Who Has the Stick.'"

11. Lyall, *Report*, 48.

12. Lyall, *Report*, 50.

13. Hota, *Violence of Recognition*, 108.

14. C. Singh, *Natural Premises*.

15. Punjab Government, *States Gazetteer of Chamba*, 222.

16. Lyall, *Report*, 39; Kapila, "Governing Morals"; Bhattacharya, "Pastoralists"; Saberwal, *Pastoral Politics*.

17. Kapila, "Governing Morals"; Kapila, "Conjugating Marriage."

18. Barnes, *Report*, 226.

19. Bhattacharya, "Pastoralists," 54; Axelby, "'It Takes Two Hands'"; Punjab Government, *Gazetteer of the Kangra District* (1926), 439.

20. Kapila, "Governing Morals," 20; see Chowdhry, *Veiled Women*; Christopher, "'Scheduled Tribe Dalit'"; Newell, "Submerged Descent Line."

21. Axelby, "'It Takes Two Hands,'" 69.

22. C. Singh, *Natural Premises*.

23. Punjab Government, *Gazetteer of the Kangra District* (1926), 439.

24. Punjab Government, *Gazetteer of the Kangra District* (1885), 150.

25. "Against the grain" is from Stoler, *Along the Archival Grain*.

26. Kapila, "Conjugating Marriage," 384, quoting NAI/Home/Public/B Proceedings/May 1879/No. 21 and NAI/Home/Public/A Proceedings/September 1879/No. 151.

27. Kapila, "Governing Morals," 127.

28. Chakravarty-Kaul, "Village Communities," 83. Processes of legal codification of property rights, and the domestic domains they structured, only intensified after Indian independence in 1947. The Land Reforms Act 1947, Panchayati Act 1951, Village Commons Land Act 1961, and Himachal Pradesh Village Common Land Utilisation Act 1974 together wiped out the unique features of customary usage and patterns of village governance.

29. See Kapila, "Governing Morals," 102–3.

30. Phillimore, "Unmarried Women."

31. Hiltebeitel, *Dharma*, 1.

32. Longkumer, *Greater India Experiment*, 8.

33. See a range of important examples in the ethnographic record, including Daftary, "Hindutva"; Longkumer, *Greater India Experiment*; Govindrajan, "Labors of Love"; and Tilche, *Adivasi Art and Activism*.

34. This is also noted by Hota, *Violence of Recognition*.

35. Bear, "Vitality of Labour."

36. Kapila, *Nullius*. Longkumer and Hota note that the renegotiation of relationships and worship practices with household, ancestral, or place-based gods is a common feature of Hindutva. Longkumer, *Greater India Experiment*; Hota, *Violence of Recognition*. While I noted this in large-scale ritual worship practices such as the Shaivite ritual practice of *nuala*, I did not note this in the worship of household gods. Instead, Gaddi people were more likely to cite that Lord Shiva was their household god and to cease daily worship of their clan god.

37. Wagner, *Gaddi Beyond Pastoralism*.

38. Parry, *Caste and Kinship*. Having good blood also spoke to concerns of caste endogamy and lineage purity.

39. Mayblin, "Untold Sacrifice," 357.

40. Snell-Rood, *No One*, 54.

41. Rashid, "Durbolota."

42. Yarris, "'Pensando mucho'"; Yarris, "'Thinking Too Much.'"

43. Han, *Life in Debt*.

44. Livingston, "Reconfiguring Old Age."

45. Cohen, "Anthropology of Senility"; Cohen, *No Aging in India*.

46. Varma, *Occupied Clinic*.

47. Govindrajan, "Labors of Love."

3. *GHAR KI TENSION*

An earlier version of some of this chapter appears in Nikita Simpson, "*Ghar ki Tension*: Domesticity and Distress in India's Aspiring Middle Class," *Journal of the Royal Anthropological Institute* 29, no. 3 (2023): 573–92.

1. Han, *Life in Debt*, 88. Han's notion of care is indebted to the ethics of acknowledgment from Stanley Cavell and Veena Das. She quotes Cavell: "We are not in, and cannot put ourselves in, the presence of characters; but it is in making their present ours, their moments as they occur, that we complete our acknowledgment of them." Cavell, *Must We Mean*, 337, quoted in Han, *Life in Debt*, 88.

2. Kapila, *Nullius*.

3. Wagner, *Gaddi Beyond Pastoralism*.

4. Kapila, "Governing Morals"; Kapila, "Conjugating Marriage."

5. Such a story resonates with existing South Asian literature on the relationship between patriarchal norms and upward social mobility. See Still, *Dalit Women*, 5–7. The Hindu model of caste-based social mobility follows a thesis of "Sanskritization," wherein the respectability of lower-caste women depends on husbands' ability to protect their wives from the advances of upper-caste men. Therein, upwardly mobile lower-caste or tribal women mimic the values of upper-caste women: adopting purdah (seclusion and veiling), restricting mobility beyond the household, and retreating from waged or agricultural work. Such literature highlights the inverse relationship between upward social mobility and female sexual liberation, where feminist scholars have argued that the intensification of capitalism in India has only made patriarchal structures of marriage, domesticity, and honor stronger and more flexible. Chowdhry, *Veiled Women*; Mies, *Lace Makers of Narsapur*.

6. Skaria, "Shades of Wildness."

7. Moodie, *We Were Adivasis*, 79.

8. Wagner, *Gaddi Beyond Pastoralism*.

9. For example, Deana Lawson, *Seagulls in the Kitchen*, 2017 (Sikkema Jenkins & Co., New York); see Simpson, "Aesthetic Politics."

10. Allerton, *Potent Landscapes*, Gammeltoft, "Domestic Moods."

11. Dickey, "Permeable Homes."

12. Alter, "Heaps of Health."

13. Donner, *Being Middle-Class.*

14. Tilche, *Adivasi Art and Activism.*

15. Banerjee, "Armed Masculinity."

16. Moodie, *We Were Adivasis*, 90–91.

17. See Aulino, *Rituals of Care.*

18. Lamb, "Making and Unmaking," 283.

19. E. V. Daniel, *Fluid Signs*, 109.

20. Gold, "Gender and Illusion."

21. Govindrajan, "Labors of Love," 213.

22. Han, *Life in Debt*, 79.

23. Streinzer, "Stretching Money."

24. Harms, "Eviction Time"; Elias and Rai, "Feminist Everyday Political Economy"; Harlan and Courtright, *Margins of Hindu Marriage*; Kapadia, *Siva and Her Sisters.* This emphasis on the domestic eternal present might be paralleled to the eternal present of the intimate conjugal bond, where the Hindu wife must retain her respectability through confinement to the household and devotion to her husband's every need.

25. I. Daniel, "Contemporary Japan."

26. Menon, "Making Śakti."

27. Harlan and Courtright, *Margins of Hindu Marriage.*

28. See Cohen, *No Aging in India*; V. Das, *Affliction*; Weaver, "Tension Among Women"; Weaver, *Sugar and Tension.*

29. As Catherine Fennell observed in her study of heat in Chicago projects. Fennell, "'Project Heat.'"

30. Gammeltoft, "Silence as a Response," 434–35.

31. Lacan, *Écrits*, 6, quoted in Gammeltoft, "Silence as a Response," 437.

32. Montoya, "Women's Sexuality"; see also Raheja and Gold, *Heron's Words*; and Wardlow, *Wayward Women.*

33. Kakar, *Shamans, Mystics, and Doctors*; Nabokov, "Expel the Lover"; Ram, *Fertile Disorder.*

34. Govindrajan, *Animal Intimacies*, 170.

35. Hollan, "Anthropology and Psychoanalysis," 158.

36. Zizek, *Sublime Object of Ideology*, 44.

37. Gammeltoft and Oosterhoff, "Mental Health," 534.

4. *FUTURE TENSION*

An earlier version of some of the ethnography in this chapter also appears in Nikita Simpson, "A Lonely Home: Balancing Intimacy and Estrangement in the Field," in *Home: Ethnographic Encounters*, ed. Johannes Lenhard and Farhan Samanani (Routledge, 2019).

1. See Marrow, "Feminine Power."

2. Jeffrey, *Timepass.* Craig Jeffrey and Constantine Nakassis also observe elsewhere that sons were seen as "exterior" to the household and only wanted to do "*time-pass*"—they would only go and use their money on their own wives—whereas daughters were seen as

"interior" to the household and more likely to care for their parents in their old age, even if they moved away in marriage. Jeffrey, *Timepass*; Nakassis, "Youth Masculinity."

3. Crapanzano, *Waiting*, 43.

4. Chua, *In Pursuit*; Chua, "Making Time."

5. Fernandes, *India's New Middle Class*.

6. Kapila, "Governing Morals"; Phillimore, "Marriage and Social Organisation."

7. Oldenberg, *Dowry Murder*.

8. Murphy, *Economization of Life*, 117.

9. Weszkalnys, "Geology, Potentiality, Speculation," 633, quoting Fortun, *Promising Genomics*, 285, and citing Røyrvik, *Allure of Capitalism*.

10. See particularly Huang, "Ambiguous Figures"; Schuster, *Social Collateral*; and Kar, "Securitizing Women."

11. Madhok and Rai, "Agency, Injury," 645.

12. Kar, "Securitizing Women."

13. Baxi, "Sexual Violence"; Baxi, *Public Secrets of Law*.

14. Berlant, *Cruel Optimism*, 199.

15. Murphy, *Economization of Life*, 114.

16. Mills, "Gendered Encounters with Modernity"; Dyson, "Friendship in Practice"; Huang, "Digital Aspirations." As women move away from the surveillance and responsibility of home for school, college, or work in factories, Aihwa Ong argues, their new experiences generate new aspirations, such as consumption practices, but these oppose traditional expectations of womanhood. See Ong, "Gender and Labour Politics," 280. The result is a form of personhood that is conflicted or divided across space and time—she calls this process "cultural struggle." The concept of cultural struggle, and its associated "split womanhood," has allowed many scholars to envision the creative forms of agency, and the new ethical positionalities, that women generated by moving across time-space.

17. For a discussion of the imaginal processes of speculation, see Bear, "Speculation."

18. Muñoz, *Cruising Utopia*, 49.

19. Muñoz, *Cruising Utopia*, 56.

20. Lester, "Inner Worlds."

21. Lester, "Inner Worlds," 2.

22. See Jassal, "Divine Politicking," for a description of the different political functions of different forms of ritual possession in the Himalayas.

23. See Sax, *God of Justice*, for an analysis of the ways in which social structures and relations within the family are contested through ritual possession; and see Nabokov, "Expel the Lover," for an analysis of the ways in which similar settings are mobilized to bolster social, and particularly patriarchal, norms.

24. V. Das, *Life and Words*.

25. Nabokov, "Expel the Lover," 299.

5. *PAGAL*

1. Sharabi, "Politics of Madness."

2. Lang, *Depression in Kerala*.

3. Luhrmann, *Of Two Minds*, 11.

4. Armstrong, *Collaborative Ethnographic Working.*

5. Biehl, *Vita.*

6. Hacking, *Mad Travelers*, 86.

7. Rubin, *Deviations*, 215–16.

8. Love, *Underdogs*, 76.

9. Love, *Underdogs*, 76.

10. Pinto, *Daughters of Parvati.*

11. Butler, *Antigone's Claim.*

12. Kapila, "Governing Morals"; Kapila, "Conjugating Marriage."

13. N. Roberts, *To Be Cared For*, 6–7.

14. See Dyson, "Adjust."

15. See Allerton, *Potent Landscapes*; and Strathern, *Gender of the Gift.*

16. Harlan and Courtright, *Margins of Hindu Marriage*, 10–11.

17. Mody, *Intimate State.*

18. See Kowalski, *Counseling Women*, for a fascinating depiction of the economy of advice that surrounds domestic and intimate partner violence in India.

19. Gahleitner found significant evidence of links between such domestic abuse and "mental tension." She highlights that such mental tension surrounded food, shelter, children's education, and, most notably, a daughter's future, abuse of children, or the effect of domestic violence on the children. Women blamed themselves for not fulfilling their responsibilities to their children when their husbands were violent. Women suffered post-traumatic stress disorder (PTSD), medically unexplained somatic illnesses such as dizziness, suicidal ideation, sleep disorders, memory and concentration loss, and dissociative symptoms. Gahleitner, *Mental Health of Survivors.*

20. Verma et al., *Report.*

21. See Mody, *Intimate State*; Grover, *Marriage, Love, Caste*; Govindrajan, "'All Cases Are False'"; and Oza, *Semiotics of Rape.*

22. See Wardlow, "Phone Friends"; and Huang, "Digital Aspirations." As Juli Huang describes of Bangladeshi young women, the mobile phone offered a means of negotiating strict gender norms without being openly transgressive. However, on the other hand, the obscurity of such intimacy led to speculation on the part of others. Huang, "Ambiguous Figures."

23. Mehtta, "Conserving Life."

24. Lamb, "Being Single in India."

25. Lester, "Back from the Edge."

26. B. Singh and Sharan, "Contagion," 458.

27. B. Singh and Sharan, "Contagion," 458.

28. Obeysekere, *Medusa's Hair.*

29. Kakar, *Shamans, Mystics, and Doctors*, 75.

30. See Simpson, "Encountering the Dain."

31. Phillimore, "Marriage and Social Organisation," 308.

32. See Munn, *Fame of Gawa*; and Graeber, *Theory of Value*, 84.

33. Munn, *Fame of Gawa*, 220.

34. Pinto, *Daughters of Parvati*, 36.

35. Doniger, *Śiva*, 223.
36. Doniger, *Śiva*, 226, 233.
37. Doniger, *Śiva*, 235.
38. Wagner, *Gaddi Beyond Pastoralism*, 45–46.
39. Pinto, *Daughters of Parvati*, 37.
40. Han, *Life in Debt*, 30.
41. Lakoff, "Simulation of Madness"; Yurchak, "Necro-Utopia," 208.

CONCLUSION

1. I have been inspired here by recent work on the ethics and politics of fieldwork from Berry et al., "Towards a Fugitive Anthropology"; Macgranahan, "Theory as Ethics"; and Günel and Watanabe, "Patchwork Ethnography."
2. Thomas, *Political Life*, 2.
3. Thomas, *Political Life*, 3.
4. See Martin, *Psychotherapy, Anthropology*.
5. See Luhrmann, *Of Two Minds*.
6. See Bemme and Béhague, "Theorising the Social."
7. Strathern, *Relations*, 2.
8. Han, *Life in Debt*, 232.
9. Strathern, *Gender of the Gift*, 12–13, quoted in Martin, *Psychotherapy, Anthropology*, 14.
10. I find Henrietta Moore's interpretation of Lacanian embodied subjectivity useful here; see Moore, *Subject of Anthropology*.
11. See Bemme and D'souza, "Global Mental Health."
12. Foucault, *Birth of the Clinic*.
13. See Armstrong, *Collaborative Ethnographic Working*, 3–4, for a cogent analysis of Foucault's application to psychiatry here.
14. For studies of psychiatric institutions and clinics, see Luhrmann, *Of Two Minds*; Pinto, *Daughters of Parvati*; Garcia, *Pastoral Clinic*; Biehl, *Vita*; and Varma, *Occupied Clinic*. For how such categories take on new meanings, see Hacking, *Mad Travelers*; Lang, *Depression in Kerala*; and Behrouzan, *Prozak Diaries*.
15. Biehl and Adams, *Arc of Interference*.
16. Case and Deaton, *Deaths of Despair*; see also Cook, *Making a Mindful Nation*.
17. See Wardell, "Naming and Framing."
18. Hecht, "Interscalar Vehicles."
19. Sophie Chao, personal communication during an "ecological distress" workshop, School of Oriental and African Studies (SOAS), University of London, May 9, 2024.
20. Todd, "Indigenous Feminist's Take," 7.
21. Haraway, "Situated Knowledges."
22. For the notion of *tension*'s scores, I am indebted to conversations with dance studies professor and choreographer Cynthia Ling Lee.

Bibliography

Agard-Jones, Vanessa. “Bodies in the System.” *Small Axe* 17, no. 3 (42) (2013): 182–92.

Ahmead, Nesar. *Khanayara Stone Quarries: A Case of Reversing the Community's Rights over Local Resources, Himachal Pradesh, India*. Artisanal and Small-Scale Mining in Asia-Pacific Case Study Series, edited by J. Jatz. Artisanal and Small-Scale Mining in Asia-Pacific Portal, 2007.

Allerton, Catherine. *Potent Landscapes: Place and Mobility in Eastern Indonesia*. Honolulu: University of Hawai'i Press, 2013.

Alter, Joseph. “Heaps of Health, Metaphysical Fitness: Ayurveda and the Ontology of Good Health in Medical Anthropology.” *Current Anthropology* 40, no. S1 (1999): S43–S66.

Arias, Daniel, Shekhar Saxena, and Stéphane Verguet. “Quantifying the Global Burden of Mental Disorders and Their Economic Value.” *eClinicalMedicine* 54, no. 101675 (2022). https://pubmed.ncbi.nlm.nih.gov/36193171/.

Armstrong, Neil. *Collaborative Ethnographic Working in Mental Health: Knowledge, Power and Hope in an Age of Bureaucratic Accountability*. London: Routledge, 2023.

Arnold, David. *Colonizing the Body: State Medicine and Epidemic Disease in Nineteenth-Century India*. Berkley: University of California Press, 1993.

Ashforth, Adam. *Witchcraft, Violence, and Democracy in South Africa*. Chicago: University of Chicago Press, 2005.

Atal, Saloni, and Juliet Foster. “‘A Woman's Life Is Tension’: A Gendered Analysis of Women's Distress in Poor Urban India.” *Transcultural Psychiatry* 58, no. 3 (2020): 404–13.

Aulino, Felicity. *Rituals of Care: Karmic Politics in an Aging Thailand*. Ithaca, NY: Cornell University Press, 2019.

Axelby, Richard. “It Takes Two Hands to Clap: How Gaddi Shepherds in the Indian Himalayas Negotiate Access to Grazing.” *Journal of Agrarian Change* 7, no. 1 (2007): 35–75.

Axelby, Richard. “Who Has the Stick Has the Buffalo: Processes of Inclusion and Exclusion on a Pasture in the Indian Himalayas.” *South Asia Multidisciplinary Academic Journal* 13 (2016): 1–16.

Banerjee, Sikata. "Armed Masculinity, Hindu Nationalism and Female Political Participation in India." *International Feminist Journal of Politics* 8, no. 1 (2006): 62–83.

Barnes, G. C. *Report of the Summary Settlement of Kangra District*. 1855. Lahore: Chronicle Press.

Baxi, Pratiksha. *Public Secrets of Law: Rape Trials in India*. Delhi: Oxford University Press, 2014.

Baxi, Pratiksha. "Sexual Violence and Its Discontents." *Annual Review of Anthropology* 43 (2014): 139–54.

Bear, Laura. "Doubt, Conflict, Mediation: The Anthropology of Modern Time." *Journal of the Royal Anthropological Institute* 20, no. S1 (2014): 3–30.

Bear, Laura. *Lines of the Nation: Indian Railway Workers, Bureaucracy, and the Intimate Historical Self*. New York: Columbia University Press, 2007.

Bear, Laura. "Speculation: A Political Economy of Technologies of Imagination." *Economy and Society* 49 (2020): 1–15.

Bear, Laura. "The Vitality of Labour and Its Ghosts." *Terrain* 69 (2018). http://journals.openedition.org/terrain/16728.

Behrouzan, Orkideh. *Prozak Diaries: Psychiatry and Generational Memory in Iran*. Stanford, CA: Stanford University Press, 2016.

Bemme, Dörte, and Dominique Béhague. "Theorising the Social in Mental Health Research and Action: A Call for More Inclusivity and Accountability." *Social Psychiatry and Psychiatric Epidemiology* 59, no. 3 (2024): 403–8.

Bemme, Dörte, and Nicole A. D'souza. "Global Mental Health and Its Discontents: An Inquiry into the Making of *Global* and *Local* Scale." *Transcultural Psychiatry* 51, no. 6 (2014): 850–74.

Berlant, Lauren. *Cruel Optimism*. Durham, NC: Duke University Press, 2011.

Berry, Maya J., Claudia Chávez Argüelles, Shanya Cordis, Sarah Ihmoud, and Elizabeth Velásquez Estrada. "Toward a Fugitive Anthropology: Gender, Race, and Violence in the Field." *Cultural Anthropology* 32, no. 4 (2017): 537–65.

Berti, Daniela. "The Local Enactment of Hindutva: Writing Stories on Local Gods in Himachal Pradesh." In *The Cultural Entrenchment of Hindutva: Local Mediations and Forms of Resistance*, edited by Daniela Berti, Nicolas Jaoul, and Pralay Kanungo, 64–69. Delhi: Routledge, 2011.

Berti, Daniela. "Possession, Communication and Power in Himachal Pradesh (North India)." In *Spirit Possession: Multidisciplinary Approaches to a Worldwide Phenomenon*, edited by Eva Pócs and András Zempléni, 1–16. Budapest: Central European University Press, 2022.

Bessire, Lucas. *Behold the Black Caiman: A Chronicle of Ayoreo Life*. Chicago: University of Chicago Press, 2014.

Bhattacharya, Neelandri. "Pastoralists in a Colonial World." In *Nature, Culture, Imperialism: Essays on Environmental History of South Asia*, edited by David Arnold and Ramachandra Guha. Delhi: Oxford University Press India, 1995.

Biehl, João G. *Vita: Life in a Zone of Social Abandonment*. Berkeley: University of California Press, 2005.

Biehl, João G., and Vincanne Adams. *Arc of Interference: Medical Anthropology for Worlds on Edge*. Durham, NC: Duke University Press, 2023.

Biehl, João G., and Amy Moran-Thomas. "Symptoms: Subjectivities, Social Ills, Technologies." *Annual Review of Anthropology* 38 (2009): 267–88.

Bindi, Serena. "Denouncing the Lack of Belief: Forms of Meta-Reflexivity About Ritual Failures in Garhwal." In *Cross-Cutting South Asian Studies: An Interdisciplinary Approach*, edited by Serena Bindi, Elena Mucciarelli, and Tiziana Pontillo, 116–44. New Delhi: DK Printworld, 2016.

Blackledge, Paul. *Marxism and Ethics: Freedom, Desire, and Revolution.* New York: SUNY Press, 2013.

Bubandt, Nils. *The Empty Seashell: Witchcraft and Doubt on an Indonesian Island.* Ithaca, NY: Cornell University Press, 2014.

Butler, Judith. *Antigone's Claim: Kinship Between Life and Death.* New York: Columbia University Press, 2002.

Campt, Tina. *Listening to Images.* Durham, NC: Duke University Press, 2017.

Case, Anne, and Angus Deaton. *Deaths of Despair and the Future of Capitalism.* Princeton, NJ: Princeton University Press, 2020.

Cavell, Stanley. *Must We Mean What We Say?* 1969. Updated ed. Cambridge: Cambridge University Press, 2002.

Chakravarty-Kaul, Minoti. "Village Communities and 'Publicness' in Northern India: Self-Governance of Common Property Resources and the Environment, 1803–2008." In *Community, Commons and Natural Resource Management in Asia*, edited by Hiroki Yanagisawa, 82–110. Singapore: NUS Press, 2015.

Chao, Sophie. *In the Shadow of the Palms: More-Than-Human Becomings in West Papua.* Durham, NC: Duke University Press, 2022.

Chowdhry, Prem. *The Veiled Women: Shifting Gender Equations in Rural Haryana.* Delhi: Oxford University Press India, 1994.

Christopher, Stephen. "Black Magic and Hali Spirituality in Himachal Pradesh." In *Mapping Identity-Induced Marginalisation in India: Inclusion and Access in the Land of Unequal Opportunities*, edited by Raosaheb K. Kale and Sanghmitra S. Acharya, 38–61. New Delhi: Springer India, 2022.

Christopher, Stephen. "'Scheduled Tribe Dalit' and the Recognition of Tribal Casteism." *Journal of Social Inclusion Studies* 6, no. 1 (2020): 7–23.

Christopher, Stephen, and Peter Phillimore. "Exploring Gaddi Pluralities: An Introduction and Overview." *HIMALAYA: The Journal of the Association for Nepal and Himalayan Studies* 42, no. 2 (2023): 3–20.

Chua, Jocelyn L. *In Pursuit of the Good Life: Aspiration and Suicide in Globalizing South India.* Berkeley: University of California Press, 2014.

Chua, Jocelyn L. "Making Time for the Children: Self-Temporalization and the Cultivation of the Antisuicidal Subject in South India." *Cultural Anthropology* 26 (2011): 112–37.

Cohen, Lawrence. *No Aging in India: Alzheimer's, the Bad Family, and Other Modern Things.* Berkeley: University of California Press, 1998.

Cohen, Lawrence. "Toward an Anthropology of Senility: Anger, Weakness, and Alzheimer's in Banaras, India." *Medical Anthropology Quarterly* 9, no. 3 (1995): 314–34.

Cook, Joanna. *Making a Mindful Nation: Mental Health and Governance in the Twenty-First Century.* Princeton, NJ: Princeton University Press, 2023.

Cooper, Timothy P. A., Michael Edwards, and Nikita Simpson. "Introduction: Back/s to the Present." In "Back to the Present," edited by Timothy P. A. Cooper, Michael Edwards, and Nikita Simpson, *American Ethnologist*, January 26, 2024. https://americanethnologist.org/online-content/collections/back-to-the-present/back-to-the-present-1/.

Crapanzano, Vincent. *Waiting: The Whites of South Africa*. New York: Random House, 1985.

Crocq, Marc-Antoine. "A History of Anxiety: From Hippocrates to DSM." *Dialogues in Clinical Neuroscience* 17, no. 3 (2015): 319–25.

Daftary, Dolly. "Hindutva, OBCs, and Koli Selfhood in Western and Central India." *Critical Asian Studies* 56, no. 1 (2023): 72–88.

Daniel, E. Valentine. *Fluid Signs: Being a Person the Tamil Way*. Berkeley: University of California Press, 1984.

Daniel, Inge. "Feeling at Home in Contemporary Japan: Space, Atmosphere and Intimacy." *Emotion, Space and Society* 15, no. 2 (2015): 47–55.

Das, Jishnu, Ranendra K. Das, and Veena Das. "The Mental Health Gender-Gap in Urban India: Patterns and Narratives." *Social Science and Medicine* 75, no. 9 (2012): 1660–72.

Das, Veena. *Affliction: Health, Disease, Poverty*. New York: Fordham University Press, 2015.

Das, Veena. *Life and Words: Violence and the Descent into the Ordinary*. Berkeley: University of California Press, 2007.

Deleuze, Gilles. "Active and Reactive." In *The New Nietzsche*, edited by David B. Allison, 80–102. Cambridge, MA: MIT Press, 1977.

Delvecchio-Good, Mary-Jo, Sandra T. Hyde, Sarah Pinto, and Byron Good. *Postcolonial Disorders*. Berkeley: University of California Press, 2008.

Denyer Willis, Laurie. "In Attention to Pain: Governance and Bodies in Brazil." *Medical Anthropology* 18, no. 39 (2020): 348–60.

Dickey, Sara. "Permeable Homes: Domestic Service, Household Space, and the Vulnerability of Class Boundaries in Urban India." *American Ethnologist* 27, no. 2 (2000): 462–89.

Dirks, Nicholas. *Castes of Mind: Colonialism and the Making of Modern India*. Princeton, NJ: Princeton University Press, 2001.

Doniger, Wendy. *Śiva, the Erotic Ascetic*. New York: Oxford University Press, 1981.

Donner, Henrike, ed. *Being Middle-Class in India: A Way of Life*. London: Routledge, 2011.

Dyson, Jane. "Adjust." *South Asia* 40, no. 2 (2017): 274–75.

Dyson, Jane. "Friendship in Practice: Girls' Work in the Indian Himalayas." *American Ethnologist* 37, no. 3 (2010): 482–98.

Elias, Juanita, and Shirin M. Rai. "Feminist Everyday Political Economy: Space, Time, and Violence." *Review of International Studies* 45, no. 2 (2019): 201–20.

Eubanks, Charlotte, and Pasang Sherpa. "We Are (Are We?) All Indigenous Here, and Other Claims About Space, Place, and Belonging in Asia." *Verge: Studies in Global Asias* 4, no. 2 (2018): vi–xiv.

Fanon, Frantz. *The Wretched of the Earth*. 1961. London: Penguin, 2001.

Fennell, Catherine. "'Project Heat' and Sensory Politics in Redeveloping Chicago Public Housing." *Ethnography* 12, no. 1 (2011): 40–64.

Fernandes, Leela. *India's New Middle Class: Democratic Politics in an Era of Economic Reform*. Minneapolis: University of Minnesota Press, 2006.

Fortun, Mike. *Promising Genomics: Iceland and deCODE Genetics in a World of Speculation*. Berkeley: University of California Press, 2008.

Foucault, Michel. *The Birth of the Clinic: An Archaeology of Medical Perception*. 1963. New York: Vintage, 1994.

Gahleitner, Edith. *Mental Health of Survivors of Domestic Violence in Rural Northern India: A Qualitative, Intersectional Approach*. ÖFSE-Forum, no. 61. Vienna: Österreichische Forschungsstiftung für Internationale Entwicklung, 2015.

Gammeltoft, Tine M. "Domestic Moods: Maternal Mental Health in Northern Vietnam." *Medical Anthropology* 37, no. 7 (2018): 1–15.

Gammeltoft, Tine M. "Silence as a Response to Everyday Violence: Understanding Domination and Distress Through the Lens of Fantasy." *Ethos* 44, no. 4 (2016): 427–47.

Gammeltoft, Tine M., and Pauline Oosterhoff. "Mental Health in Domestic Worlds." *Medical Anthropology* 37, no. 7 (2018): 533–37.

Garcia, Angela. *The Pastoral Clinic: Addiction and Dispossession Along the Rio Grande*. Berkeley: University of California Press, 2010.

GD Mental Disorders Collaborators. "Global, Regional, and National Burden of 12 Mental Disorders in 204 Countries and Territories, 1990–2019: A Systematic Analysis for the Global Burden of Disease Study 2019." *Lancet Psychiatry* 9, no. 2 (2019): 137–50.

Geschiere, Peter. *The Modernity of Witchcraft: Politics and the Occult in Postcolonial Africa*. Charlottesville: University Press of Virginia, 1997.

Geschiere, Peter. "Witchcraft as the Dark Side of Kinship: Dilemmas of Social Security in New Contexts." *Etnofoor* 16, no. 1 (2003): 43–61.

Gilroy, Paul. *The Black Atlantic*. 1995. London: Verso Books, 2022.

Gold, Ann G. "Gender and Illusion in a Rajasthani Yogic Tradition." In *Gender, Genre, and Power in South Asian Expressive Traditions*, edited by Arjun Appadurai, Frank J. Korom, and Margaret A. Mills, 102–36. Philadelphia: University of Pennsylvania Press, 1991.

Good, Byron J. "The Heart of What's the Matter: The Semantics of Illness in Iran." *Culture, Medicine, Psychiatry* 1, no. 1 (1977): 25–58.

Govindrajan, Radhika. "'All Cases Are False': Law, Gendered Violence, and the Politics of Thickening in Himalayan India." *Journal of the Royal Anthropological Institute* 31 (2024): 198–216.

Govindrajan, Radhika. *Animal Intimacies: Interspecies Relatedness in India's Central Himalayas*. Chicago: University of Chicago Press, 2018.

Govindrajan, Radhika. "Labors of Love: On the Political Economies and Ethics of Bovine Politics in Himalayan India." *Cultural Anthropology* 36, no. 2 (2021): 193–221.

Graeber, David. *Toward an Anthropological Theory of Value: The False Coin of Our Own Dreams*. New York: Palgrave, 2001.

Grover, Shalini. *Marriage, Love, Caste and Kinship Support: Lived Experiences of the Urban Poor in India*. New Delhi: Social Science Press, 2011.

Günel, Gökçe, and Chika Watanabe. "Patchwork Ethnography." *American Ethnologist* 51, no. 1 (2023): 131–39.

Guru, Gopal. *Humiliation: Claims and Context*. Oxford: Oxford University Press, 2009.

Hacking, Ian. *Mad Travelers: Reflections on the Reality of Transient Mental Illnesses*. Charlottesville: University Press of Virginia, 1998.

Halliburton, Murphy. "'Just Some Spirits': The Erosion of Spirit Possession and the Rise of 'Tension' in South India." *Medical Anthropology* 24, no. 2 (2005): 111–44.

Han, Clara. *Life in Debt: Times of Care and Violence in Neoliberal Chile*. Berkeley: University of California Press, 2012.

Haraway, Donna. "Situated Knowledges: The Science Question in Feminism and the Privilege of Partial Perspective." *Feminist Studies* 14, no. 3 (1988): 575–99.

Harlan, Lindsey, and Paul B. Courtright, eds. *From the Margins of Hindu Marriage: Essays on Gender, Religion, and Culture*. New York: Oxford University Press, 1995.

Harms, Erik. "Eviction Time in the New Saigon: Temporalities of Displacement in the Rubble of Development." *Cultural Anthropology* 28, no. 2 (2013): 344–68.

Hecht, Gabrielle. "Interscalar Vehicles for an African Anthropocene: On Waste, Temporality, and Violence." *Cultural Anthropology* 33, no. 1 (2018): 109–41.

Hiltebeitel, Alf. *Dharma: Its Early History in Law, Religion, and Narrative*. Honolulu: University of Hawai'i Press, 2010.

Hollan, Douglas. "Anthropology and Psychoanalysis: The Looping Effects of People and Social Worlds." *Annual Review of Anthropology* 51, no. 1 (2022): 155–71.

Hota, Pinky. *The Violence of Recognition: Adivasi Indigeneity and Anti-Dalitness in India*. Philadelphia: University of Pennsylvania Press, 2023.

Huang, Juli. "The Ambiguous Figures of Social Enterprise: Gendered Flexibility and Relational Work Among the iAgents of Bangladesh." *American Ethnologist* 44 (2017): 603–16.

Huang, Juli. "Digital Aspirations: 'Wrong-Number' Mobile-Phone Relationships and Experimental Ethics Among Women Entrepreneurs in Rural Bangladesh." *Journal of the Royal Anthropological Institute* 24 (2018): 107–25.

Hughes, Geoff, Megnaa Mehtta, Chiara Bresciani, and Stuart Strange. "Introduction: Ugly Emotions and the Politics of Accusation." *Cambridge Journal of Anthropology* 37, no. 2 (2019): 1–20.

Hunter, William W. *The Imperial Gazetteer of India*. Vol. 11. Oxford: Clarendon, 1908.

Jadhav, Sushrut. "The Cultural Origins of Western Depression." *International Journal of Social Psychiatry* 42, no. 4 (1996): 269–86.

Jassal, Aftab Singh. "Divine Politicking: A Rhetorical Approach to Deity Possession in the Himalayas." *Religions* 7, no. 9 (2016): 117. https://doi.org/10.3390/rel7090117.

Jeffrey, Craig. *Timepass: Youth, Class, and the Politics of Waiting in India*. Stanford, CA: Stanford University Press, 2010.

Kaiser, Bonnie, and Lesley Jo Weaver. "Culture-Bound Syndromes, Idioms of Distress, and Cultural Concepts of Distress: New Directions for an Old Concept in Psychological Anthropology." *Transcultural Psychiatry* 56, no. 4 (2019): 589–98.

Kakar, Sudhir. *Shamans, Mystics, and Doctors: A Psychological Inquiry into India and Its Healing Traditions*. New York: Knopf, 1982.

Kapadia, Karin. *Siva and Her Sisters: Gender, Caste, and Class in Rural South India*. Boulder, CO: Westview, 1995.

Kapila, Kriti. "Conjugating Marriage: State Legislation and Gaddi Kinship." *Contributions to Indian Sociology* 38, no. 3 (2004): 379–409.

Kapila, Kriti. "Governing Morals: State, Marriage and Household Amongst the Gaddis of North India." PhD diss., London School of Economics, 2003. http://etheses.lse.ac.uk/id/eprint/2881.

Kapila, Kriti. "The Measure of a Tribe: The Cultural Politics of Constitutional Reclassification in North India." *Journal of the Royal Anthropological Institute* 14, no. 1 (2008): 117–34.

Kapila, Kriti. *Nullius: The Anthropology of Ownership, Sovereignty and the Law in India.* London: HAU Books, 2022.

Kar, Sohini. "Securitizing Women: Gender, Precaution, and Risk in Indian Finance." *Signs: Journal of Women in Culture and Society* 43, no. 2 (2018): 301–25.

Kermode, Michelle, Helen Herrman, Ranjanikant Arole, Joshua White, Ramaswamy Premkumar, and Vikram Patel. "Empowerment of Women and Mental Health Promotion: A Qualitative Study in Rural Maharashtra, India." *BMC Public Health* 7 (2007): 1–10.

Khera, Dipti. *The Place of Many Moods: Udaipur's Painted Lands and India's Eighteenth Century.* Princeton, NJ: Princeton University Press, 2020.

Kleinman, Arthur. "Anthropology and Psychiatry: The Role of Culture in Cross-Cultural Research on Illness." *British Journal of Psychiatry* 151 (1987): 447–54.

Kowalski, Julia. *Counseling Women: Kinship Against Violence in India.* Philadelphia: University of Pennsylvania Press, 2022.

Lacan, Jacques. *Écrits.* Translated by Bruce Fink in collaboration with Héloise Fink and Russell Grigg. 1966. New York: W. W. Norton, 2006.

Lakoff, Andrew. "The Simulation of Madness: Buenos Aires, 1903." *Critical Inquiry* 31, no. 4 (2005): 848–73.

Lamb, Sarah. "Being Single in India: Gendered Identities, Class Mobilities, and Personhoods in Flux." *Ethos* 46, no. 1 (2018): 49–69.

Lamb, Sarah. "The Making and Unmaking of Persons: Notes on Aging and Gender in North India." *Ethos* 25, no. 3 (1997): 279–302.

Lamb, Sarah. *White Saris and Sweet Mangoes: Aging, Gender, and Body in North India.* Berkeley: University of California Press, 2000.

Lang, Claudia. *Depression in Kerala: Ayurveda and Mental Health Care in 21st Century India.* London: Routledge, 2018.

Lester, Rebecca J. "Back from the Edge of Existence: A Critical Anthropology of Trauma." *Transcultural Psychiatry* 50, no. 5 (2013): 753–62.

Lester, Rebecca J. "Inner Worlds as Social Systems: How Insights from Anthropology Can Inform Clinical Practice." *Social Science and Medicine—Mental Health* 2 (2022): 100068. https://doi.org/10.1016/j.ssmmh.2022.100068.

Livingston, Julie. 2003. "Reconfiguring Old Age: Elderly Women and Concerns over Care in Southeastern Botswana." *Medical Anthropology* 22, no. 3 (2003): 205–31.

Longkumer, Arkotong. *The Greater India Experiment: Hindutva and the Northeast.* Stanford, CA: Stanford University Press, 2020.

Love, Heather. *Underdogs: Social Deviance and Queer Theory.* Chicago: University of Chicago Press, 2021.

Luhrmann, Tanya M. *Of Two Minds: The Growing Disorder in American Psychiatry*. New York: Knopf, 2000.

Lyall, James B. *Report of the Land Revenue Settlement of Kangra District, 1865–72*. Lahore: Central Jail Press, 1874. https://hpkangra.nic.in/document-category/land-revenue-settlement-en/.

Macdonald, Helen. *Witchcraft Accusations in Central India: The Fragmented Urn*. Oxford: Routledge, 2020.

Macgranahan, Carole. "Theory as Ethics." *American Ethnologist* 49, no. 3 (2022): 289–301.

Madhok, Sumi, and Shirin M. Rai. "Agency, Injury and Transgressive Politics in Neoliberal Times." *Signs* 37 (2012): 645–69.

Marriott, McKim. "The Female Family Core Explored Ethnosociologically." *Contributions to Indian Sociology* 32, no. 2 (1998): 279–304.

Marriott, McKim. *Hindu Transactions: Diversity Without Dualism*. Chicago: University of Chicago Press, 1976.

Marrow, Jocelyn. "Feminine Power or Feminine Weakness? North Indian Girls' Struggles with Aspirations, Agency, and Psychosomatic Illness." *American Ethnologist* 40, no. 2 (2013): 347–61.

Marsilli-Vargas, Xochitl. *Genres of Listening: An Ethnography of Psychoanalysis in Buenos Aries*. Durham, NC: Duke University Press, 2022.

Martin, Keir, ed. *Psychotherapy, Anthropology and the Work of Culture*. Oxford: Routledge, 2019.

Mayblin, Maya. "The Untold Sacrifice: The Monotony and Incompleteness of Self-Sacrifice in Northeast Brazil." *Ethnos* 79, no. 3 (2014): 342–64.

Mehtta, Megnaa. "Conserving Life: Forest Imaginaries and Competing Values in the Sundarbans Forests of India." PhD diss., London School of Economics and Political Science, 2019.

Menon, Usha. "Making Śakti: Controlling (Natural) Impurity for Female (Cultural) Power." *Ethos* 30, nos. 1–2 (2002): 140–57.

Mies, Maria. *The Lace Makers of Narsapur: Indian Housewives Produce for the World Market*. London: Zed Books, 1982.

Mills, Mary-Beth. "Gendered Encounters with Modernity: Labor Migrants and Marriage Choices in Contemporary Thailand." *Identities* 5, no. 3 (1998): 301–34.

Mody, Perveez. *The Intimate State: Love-Marriage and the Law in Delhi*. New Delhi: Routledge, 2008.

Montoya, Rosario. "Women's Sexuality, Knowledge, and Agency in Rural Nicaragua." In *Gender's Place: Feminist Anthropologies of Latin America*, edited by Rosario Montoya, Lessie Jo Frazier, and Janise Hurtig, 65–88. New York: Palgrave Macmillan, 2002.

Moodie, Megan. *We Were Adivasis: Aspiration in an Indian Scheduled Tribe*. Chicago: University of Chicago Press, 2015.

Moore, Henrietta. *The Subject of Anthropology: Gender, Symbolism and Psychoanalysis*. Cambridge, UK: Polity, 2007.

Mosse, David, Sushrut Jadhav, and Ned Dostaler. "Minds of Caste—Discrimination and Its Affects." *Anthropology Today* 32, no. 1 (2016): 1–2.

Munn, Nancy. *The Fame of Gawa: A Symbolic Study of Value Transformation in Massim Society*. Durham, NC: Duke University Press, 1986.

Muñoz, José Esteban. *Cruising Utopia: The Then and There of Queer Futurity*. New York: New York University Press, 2009.

Murphy, Michelle. *The Economization of Life*. Durham, NC: Duke University Press, 2017.

Nabokov, Isabelle. "Expel the Lover, Recover the Wife: Symbolic Analysis of a South Indian Exorcism." *Journal of the Royal Anthropological Institute* 3, no. 2 (1997): 297–316.

Nakassis, Constantine V. "Youth Masculinity, 'Style' and the Peer Group in Tamil Nadu, India." *Contributions to Indian Sociology* 47, no. 2 (2013): 245–69.

Narayan, Kirin. *Mondays on the Dark Night of the Moon: Himalayan Foothill Folktales*. In collaboration with Urmila Devi Sood. Oxford: Oxford University Press, 1997.

Newell, William H. "The Submerged Descent Line Among the Gaddi People of North India." *Journal of the Royal Anthropological Institute* 92, no. 1 (1962): 13–22.

Ngai, Sianne. *Ugly Feelings*. Cambridge, MA: Harvard University Press, 2007.

Nichter, Mark. "Idioms of Distress: Alternatives in the Expression of Psychosocial Distress; a Case Study from South India." *Culture, Medicine, Psychiatry* 5, no. 4 (1981): 379–408.

Nichter, Mark. "Idioms of Distress Revisited." *Culture, Medicine, Psychiatry* 34, no. 2 (2010): 401–16.

Obeysekere, Gananath. *Medusa's Hair: An Essay on Personal Symbols and Religious Experience*. Chicago: University of Chicago Press, 1981.

Oldenberg, Veena T. *Dowry Murder: The Imperial Origins of a Cultural Crime*. Oxford: Oxford University Press, 2002.

Ong, Aihwa. "The Gender and Labor Politics of Postmodernity." *Annual Review of Anthropology* 20 (1991): 279–309.

Oza, Rupa. *Semiotics of Rape: Sexual Subjectivity and Violation in Rural India*. Durham, NC: Duke University Press, 2022.

Paralikar, Vasudeo, Mohan Agashe, Sanjeev Sarmukaddam, Shamishtha Deshpande, Vejaya Goyal, and Mitchell G. Weiss. "Cultural Epidemiology of Neurasthenia Spectrum Disorders in Four General Hospital Outpatient Clinics of Urban Pune, India." *Transcultural Psychiatry* 48, no. 3 (2011): 257–83.

Parry, Jonathan. *Caste and Kinship in Kangra*. London: Routledge and Kegan Paul, 1979.

Parry, Jonathan. *Classes of Labour: Work and Life in a Central Indian Steel Town*. London: Routledge and Kegan Paul, 2020.

Patel, Vikram, and Nandini Oomman. "Mental Health Matters Too: Gynaecological Symptoms and Depression in South Asia." *Reproductive Health Matters* 7, no. 14 (1999): 30–38.

Patel, Vikram, Jerson Pereira, Livia Countinho, Romaldina Fernandes, John Fernandes, and Antony Mann. "Poverty, Psychological Disorder and Disability in Primary Care Attenders in Goa, India." *British Journal of Psychiatry* 172, no. 6 (1998): 533–36.

Phillimore, Peter. "Marriage and Social Organisation Among Pastoralists of the Dhaula Dhar." PhD diss., University of Durham, 1982.

Phillimore, Peter. "'That Used to Be a Famous Village': Shedding the Past in Rural North India." *Modern Asian Studies* 48, no. 1 (2014): 159–87.

Phillimore, Peter. "Unmarried Women of the Dhaula Dhar: Celibacy and Social Control in Northwest India." *Journal of Anthropological Research* 47, no. 3 (1991): 331–50.

Pinney, Chris. "On Living in the Kal(i)yug: Notes from Nagda, Madhya Pradesh." *Contributions to Indian Sociology* 33, nos. 1–2 (1999): 77–106.

Pinto, Sarah. *Daughters of Parvati: Women and Madness in Contemporary India*. Philadelphia: University of Pennsylvania Press, 2014.

Punjab Government. *Gazetteer of the Kangra District*. Lahore: Government Press, 1885.

Punjab Government. *Gazetteer of the Kangra District*. Lahore: Government Press, 1926.

Punjab Government. *States Gazetteer of Chamba District*. Lahore: Government Press, 1904.

Qureshi, Kaveri. *Chronic Illness in a Pakistani Labour Diaspora*. Durham, NC: Carolina Academic Press, 2019.

Rabinbach, Anson. *The Human Motor: Energy, Fatigue, and the Origins of Modernity*. Berkeley: University of California Press, 1990.

Raheja, Gloria G., and Ann G. Gold. *Listen to the Heron's Words: Reimagining Gender and Kinship in North India*. Berkeley: University of California Press, 1994.

Ram, Kalpana. *Fertile Disorder: Spirit Possession and Its Provocation of the Modern*. Honolulu: University of Hawai'i Press, 2013.

Ramaswami, Shankar. "Masculinity, Respect, and the Tragic: Themes of Proletarian Humor in Contemporary Industrial Delhi." *International Review of Social History* 51, no. S41 (2006): 203–27.

Rashid, Sabina. "Durbolota (Weakness), Chinta rog (Worry Illness), and Poverty: Explanations of White Discharge Among Married Adolescent Women in an Urban Slum in Dhaka, Bangladesh." *Medical Anthropology Quarterly* 21 (2007): 108–32.

Roberts, Nathaniel. *To Be Cared For: The Power of Conversion and the Foreignness of Belonging in an Indian Slum*. Berkeley: University of California Press, 2016.

Roberts, Tessa, Ritu Shrivastava, Mirja Koschorke, Vikram Patel, Rahul Shidhaye, and Sujit D. Rathod. "Is There a Medicine for These Tensions? Barriers to Treatment-Seeking for Depressive Symptoms in Rural India: A Qualitative Study." *Social Science and Medicine* 246 (2020): 112741. https://pubmed.ncbi.nlm.nih.gov/31918347/.

Rodrigues, Merlyn, Vikram Patel, Surinder Jaswal, and Nandita de Souza. "Listening to Mothers: Qualitative Studies on Motherhood and Depression from Goa, India." *Social Science and Medicine* 57, no. 10 (2003): 1797–806.

Rose, Horace A. *A Glossary of the Tribes and Castes of the Punjab and North-West Frontier Province*. Lahore: Government Publishing, Punjab, 1919.

Røyrvik, Emil A. *The Allure of Capitalism: An Ethnography of Management and the Global Economy in Crisis*. Oxford: Berghahn, 2011.

Rubin, Gayle. *Deviations: A Gayle Rubin Reader*. Durham, NC: Duke University Press, 2011.

Rutherford, Danilyn. "Affect Theory and the Empirical." *Annual Review of Anthropology* 45 (2016): 285–300.

Saberwal, Vasant. *Pastoral Politics: Shepherds, Bureaucrats, and Conservation in the Western Himalaya*. Delhi: Oxford University Press, 1999.

Sax, William. *God of Justice: Ritual Healing and Social Justice in the Central Himalayas.* Oxford: Oxford University Press, 2009.

Scarry, Elaine. *The Body in Pain: The Making and Unmaking of the World.* Oxford: Oxford University Press, 1985.

Schnegg, Michael. "Collective Loneliness: Theorizing Emotions as Atmospheres." *Current Anthropology* 66, no. 2 (2025): 206–31.

Schuster, Caroline E. *Social Collateral: Women and Microfinance in Paraguay's Smuggling Economy.* Oakland: University of California Press, 2015.

Scott, Darieck. *Extravagant Abjection: Blackness, Power, and Sexuality in the African American Literary Imagination.* New York: NYU Press, 2010.

Shah, Alpa, and Jens Lerche. *Ground Down by Growth: Tribe, Caste, Class and Inequality in Twenty-First-Century India.* London: Pluto, 2017.

Sharabi, Asaf. "The Politics of Madness and Spirit Possession in Northern India." *Medical Anthropology* 40, no. 2 (2020): 182–95.

Sharma, Mahesh. "Ritual, Performance, and Transmission: The Gaddi Shepherds of Himachal Himalayas." *Oral Tradition* 29, no. 2 (2015): 271–90.

Sharma, Mahesh. "Symbols of Empowerment: Possession, Ritual and Healers in Himachal Himalaya (North India)." *Journal of Asian and African Studies* 45, no. 2 (2010): 196–208.

Shidhaye, Rahul, and Vikram Patel. "Association of Socio-Economic, Gender and Health Factors with Common Mental Disorders in Women: A Population-Based Study of 5703 Married Rural Women in India." *International Journal of Epidemiology* 39, no. 6 (2010): 1510–21.

Simpson, Nikita. "Aesthetic Politics in Contemporary India." *Focaal* 2023, no. 95 (2023): 113–19.

Simpson, Nikita. "Encountering the Dain: Space-Time, Witchcraft Anxiety, and Gaddi Tribal Belonging." *HIMALAYA: The Journal of the Association for Nepal and Himalayan Studies* 42, no. 2 (2023): 70–85.

Simpson, Nikita. "*Ghar ki Tension*: Domesticity and Distress in India's Aspiring Middle Class." *Journal of the Royal Anthropological Institute* 29, no. 3 (2023): 573–92.

Simpson, Nikita. "*Kamzori*: Aging, Care and Alienation in the Post-Pastoral Himalaya." *Medical Anthropology Quarterly* 36, no. 3 (2022): 391–411.

Simpson, Nikita. "A Lonely Home: Balancing Intimacy and Estrangement in the Field." In *Home: Ethnographic Encounters*, edited by Johannes Lenhard and Farhan Samanani. Routledge, 2019.

Singh, Bhrigupati. "Anthropological Investigations of Vitality: Life Force as a Dimension Distinct from Time and Space." *HAU: Journal of Ethnographic Theory* 8, no. 3 (2018): 550–65.

Singh, Bhrigupati. "Can a Neighborhood Fall Sick? Opioid Addiction, Collective Violence and Currents of Death in Contemporary India." *Medical Anthropology Quarterly* 35, no. 2 (2021): 159–89.

Singh, Bhrigupati, and Pratap Sharan. "The Contagion of Mental Illness: Insights from a Sufi Shrine." *Transcultural Psychiatry* 60, no. 3 (2023): 457–75.

Singh, Chetan. *Natural Premises: Ecology and Peasant Life in the Western Himalaya, 1800–1950.* Delhi: Oxford University Press India, 1998.

Skaria, Ajay. "Shades of Wildness: Tribe, Caste, and Gender in Western India." *Journal of Asian Studies* 56, no. 3 (1997): 726–45.

Skaria, Ajay. "Women, Witchcraft and Gratuitous Violence in Colonial Western India." *Past and Present* 155, no. 1 (1997): 109–41.

Snell-Rood, Claire. *No One Will Let Her Live: Women's Struggle for Well-Being in a Delhi Slum*. Berkeley: University of California Press, 2015.

Still, Clarinda. *Dalit Women: Honour and Patriarchy in South India.* London: Routledge, 2014.

Stoler, Ann Laura. *Along the Archival Grain: Epistemic Anxieties and Colonial Common Sense.* Princeton, NJ: Princeton University Press, 2008.

Stoler, Ann Laura. "Making Empire Respectable: The Politics of Race and Sexual Morality in 20th-Century Colonial Cultures." *American Ethnologist* 16, no. 4 (1989): 634–60.

Strathern, Marilyn. *The Gender of the Gift: Problems with Women and Problems with Society in Melanesia.* Berkeley: University of California Press, 1988.

Strathern, Marilyn. *Relations: An Anthropological Account*. Durham, NC: Duke University Press, 2020.

Streinzer, Andreas. "Stretching Money to Pay the Bills: The Temporal Modalities and Relational Practices of Getting By in the Greek Economic Crisis." *Cambridge Journal of Anthropology* 34, no. 1 (2016): 45–57.

Thomas, Deborah. *Political Life in the Wake of the Plantation: Soverignty, Witnessing, Repair*. Durham, NC: Duke University Press, 2019.

Tilche, Alice. *Adivasi Art and Activism: Curation in a Nationalist Age.* Seattle: University of Washington Press, 2022.

Todd, Zoe. "An Indigenous Feminist's Take on the Ontological Turn: 'Ontology' Is Just Another Word for Colonialism." *Journal of Historical Sociology* 29, no. 1 (2016): 4–22.

Trawick, Margaret. *Notes on Love in a Tamil Family.* Berkeley: University of California Press, 1990.

Tsing, Anna Lowenhaupt, Andrew S. Mathews, and Nils Bubandt. "Patchy Anthropocene: Landscape Structure, Multispecies History, and the Retooling of Anthropology: An Introduction to Supplement 20." *Current Anthropology* 60, no. S20 (2019): S186–S197.

Varma, Saiba. *The Occupied Clinic: Militarism and Care in Kashmir*. Durham, NC: Duke University Press, 2020.

Venkat, Bharat J. *At the Limits of Cure.* Durham, NC: Duke University Press, 2021.

Verma, Jagdish Sharan, Leila Seth, and Gopal Subramanian. *Report of the Committee on Amendments to Criminal Law*. New Delhi: Government of India, 2013.

Wadley, Susan. "No Longer a Wife: Widows in Rural North India." In *From the Margins of Hindu Marriage: Essays on Gender, Religion, and Culture*, edited by Lindsey Harlan and Paul B. Courtright, 92–118. New York: Oxford University Press, 1995.

Wadley, Susan. *Shakti: Power in the Conceptual Structure of Karimpur Religion*. Chicago: University of Chicago Press, 1975.

Wagner, Anya. *The Gaddi Beyond Pastoralism: Making Place in the Indian Himalayas.* Oxford: Berghahn Books, 2013.

Wardell, Susan. *Living in the Tension: Care, Selfhood, and Wellbeing Among Faith-Based Youth Workers*. Durham, NC: Carolina Academic Press, 2018.

Wardell, Susan. "Naming and Framing Ecological Distress." *Medicine Anthropology Theory* 7, no. 2 (2020): 187–201.
Wardlow, Holly. "HIV, Phone Friends and Affective Technology in Papua New Guinea." In *The Moral Economy of Mobile Phones: Pacific Islands Perspectives*, edited by Robert J. Foster and Heather A. Horst, 39–52. Canberra: ANU Press, 2018.
Wardlow, Holly. *Wayward Women: Sexuality and Agency in a New Guinea Society*. Berkeley: University of California Press, 2006.
Weaver, Lesley Jo. *Sugar and Tension: Diabetes and Gender in Modern India.* New Brunswick, NJ: Rutgers University Press, 2018.
Weaver, Lesley Jo. "Tension Among Women in North India: An Idiom of Distress and a Cultural Syndrome." *Culture, Medicine, Psychiatry* 41, no. 1 (2017): 35–55.
Weszkalnys, Gisa. "Geology, Potentiality, Speculation: On the Indeterminacy of First Oil." *Cultural Anthropology* 30, no. 4 (2015): 611–39.
Wilson, Elizabeth A. *Gut Feminism.* Durham, NC: Duke University Press, 2015.
Xaxa, Virginius. *State, Society and Tribes: Issues in Post-Colonial India.* London: Pearson, 2008.
Yarris, Kristin. "The Pain of 'Thinking Too Much': Dolor de Cerebro and the Embodiment of Social Hardship Among Nicaraguan Women." *Ethos* 39, no. 2 (2011): 226–48.
Yarris, Kristin. "'Pensando Mucho' ('Thinking Too Much'): Embodied Distress Among Grandmothers in Nicaraguan Transnational Families." *Culture, Medicine, Psychiatry* 38, no. 3 (2014): 473–98.
Yurchak, Alexei. "Necro-Utopia: The Politics of Indistinction and the Aesthetics of the Non-Soviet." *Current Anthropology* 49, no. 2 (2008): 199–224.
Žižek, Slavoj. *The Sublime Object of Ideology.* London: Verso Books, 1989.

Index

www.ingramcontent.com/pod-product-compliance
Lightning Source LLC
Chambersburg PA
CBHW030315270326
41926CB00010B/1368

* 9 7 8 1 4 7 8 0 3 3 2 9 5 *